Ernst Schering Research Foundation Workshop 47
Neuroinflammation in Stroke

Springer
Berlin
Heidelberg
New York
Hong Kong
London
Milan
Paris
Tokyo

Ernst Schering Research Foundation
Workshop 47

Neuroinflammation in Stroke

U. Dirnagl, B. Elger
Editors

With 30 Figures and 9 Tables

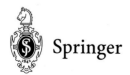 Springer

Series Editors: G. Stock and M. Lessl

ISSN 0947-6075
ISBN 3-540-40348-5 Springer-Verlag Berlin Heidelberg New York

Library of Congress Cataloging-in-Publication Data
Neuroinflammation in stroke / U. Dirnagl and B. Elger, editors.
   p.; cm. – (Ernst Schering Research Foundation workshop, ISSN 0947-6075; 47)
   Includes bibliographical references and index.
   ISBN 3-540-40348-5 (alk. paper)
   1. Cerebrovascular disease. 2. Cerebral ischemia. 3. Inflammation. I. Dirnagl, Ulrich. II.
Elger, B. (Bernd), 1955– III. Series.
   [DNLM: 1. Cerebrovascular Accident–physiopathology. 2. Cerebrovascular
Accident–drug therapy. WL 355 N49445 2004]
   RC388.5.N463 2004
   616.8'1–dc 22

Springer-Verlag is a part of Springer Science+Business Media

springeronline.com

© Springer-Verlag Berlin · Heidelberg 2004
Printed in Germany

Typesetting: K+V Fotosatz GmbH, Beerfelden

Cover design: design & production GmbH, Heidelberg

21/3130/AG-5 4 3 2 1 0 – Printed on acid-free paper

Preface

Stroke is a major cause of death and disability in industrialized countries. To date, the medical need of efficient therapy for this devastating cerebrovascular disorder remains unmet. During the last decades, the development of pharmacological stroke therapies was aimed at improving patient outcome by restoration of cerebral blood flow or protection from acute neuronal cell death. Almost all of

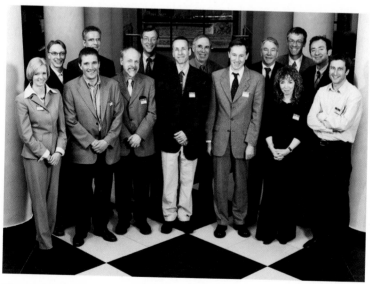

The participants of the workshop

these approaches targeted the very early events after vascular occlusion. However, primarily for logistical reasons, only a small portion of strokes can be treated within 6–10 h after the insult.

In recent years it has been recognized that stroke pathophysiology is a dynamic process, and that delayed processes, which occur during the days and weeks following arterial occlusion, may lead to further deterioration or to impairment of recovery and rehabilitation in subacute and chronic stages. Evidence is accumulating that neuroinflammation is a major player in these delayed pathophysiological processes. While some components of neuroinflammation such as removal of cell debris and release of trophic factors may support recovery processes, others such as the generation of free radicals and other cytotoxic mediators are deleterious for brain tissue after ischemia. Thus, neuroinflammation after stroke can be considered a double-edged sword, having potentially both detrimental and beneficial effects. As in other inflammatory reactions in the body, the cellular and humoral interactions are highly complex in the setting of neuroinflammation. Knowledge in this rather new field of research is rapidly growing. It is becoming evident that neuroinflammation is a promising target for novel therapeutic approaches to improve outcome after stroke. Hence, it was the intention of the workshop "Neuroinflammation in Stroke" to review basic stroke pathomechanisms, to identify possible targets for pharmacological interventions, and to consider the feasibility of conducting successful clinical stroke trials using anti-inflammatory or inflammation-modulating compounds.

U. Dirnagl, B. Elger

Contents

List of Editors and Contributors

Editors

Dirnagl, U.
Abteilung Experimentelle Neurologie, Charité, Humboldt University,
Schumannstrasse 20/21, 10098 Berlin, Germany
e-mail: ulrich.dirnagl@charite.de

Elger, B.
Neurology Research, Schering AG, Müllerstr. 178, 13342 Berlin,
Germany
e-mail: bernd.elger@schering.de

Contributors

Allan, S.
School of Biological Sciences, University of Manchester,
Oxford Road, Manchester, M13 9PT, UK
e-mail: stuart.allan@man.ac.uk

Becker, K.
Department of Neurology, Box 359775, Harborview Medical Center,
325 Ninth Avenue, Seattle, WA 98104-2499, USA
e-mail: Kjb@u.washington.edu

van Beek, J.
H. Lundbeck A7S, Molecular Disease Biology (807), Ottiliavej 7,
2500 Valby, Denmark
e-mail: JVBE@lundbeck.com

Chamorro, A.
Hospital Clinic, Clinical Institute of Nervous System Diseases,
Institut Investigations Biomedicas August Pi i Sunyer (IDIBAPS),
Barcelona, Spain
e-mail: chamorro@medicina.ub.es

Dirnagl, U.
Abteilung Experimentelle Neurologie, Charité, Humboldt University,
Schumannstrasse 20/21, 10098 Berlin, Germany
e-mail: ulrich.dirnagl@charite.de

Engelhardt, B.
Max Planck Institute for Vascular Biology, ZMBE,
Von Esmarch-Straße 56, 48149, Münster, Germany
e-mail: bengel@mpi-muenster.mpg.de

Hacke, W.
Department of Neurology, University of Heidelberg,
Im Neuenheimer Feld 400, 69120 Heidelberg, Germany

Hallenbeck, J.
Stroke Branch, NINDS, NIH, Bldg. 36, Room 4A03,
36 Convent Drive, MSC 4128, Bethesda, MD, 20892-4128, USA
e-mail: Hallenbj@ninds.nih.gov

Kauppinen, T.
A.I. Virtanen Institute for Molecular Sciences, University of Kuopio,
Neulaniementie 2, 70210 Kuopio, Finland

Koistinaho, J.
A.I. Virtanen Institute for Molecular Sciences, University of Kuopio,
Neulaniementie 2, 70210 Kuopio, Finland
e-mail: Jari.Koistinaho@uku.fi

Koistinaho, M.
A.I. Virtanen Institute for Molecular Sciences, University of Kuopio,
Neulaniementie 2, 70210 Kuopio, Finland

McCarron, R.
Resuscitative Medicine Department, NMRC, Code 032,
503 Robert Grant Ave., Silver Spring, MD, 20910-7500, USA
e-mail: McCarronR@nnmc.navy.mil

Mun-Bryce, S.
Department of Neurology, Neuroscience,
Cell Biology and Physiology, University of New Mexico Health
Sciences Center, Albuquerque, NM 87131, USA
e-mail: SMun-bryce@salud.unm.edu

Planas, A.M.
Department of Pharmacology and Toxicology, Institut Investigations
Biomédicas – Consejo Superior Investigaciones Cientificas,
Barcelona, Spain

Ringleb, P.
Department of Neurology, University of Heidelberg,
Im Neuenheimer Feld 400, 69120 Heidelberg, Germany

Rosenberg, G.A.
Health Sciences Center, Department of Neurology MSC10 51450,
1 University of New Mexico, Albuquerque, NM 87131, USA
e-mail: grosenberg@salud.unm.edu

Ruetzler, C.
Stroke Branch, NINDS, NIH, Bldg. 36, Room 4A03,
36 Convent Drive, MSC 4128, Bethesda, MD, 20892-4128, USA
e-mail: Ruetzlec@ninds.nih.gov

Schwaninger, M.
Department of Neurology, University of Heidelberg,
Im Neuenheimer Feld 400, 69120 Heidelberg, Germany
e-mail: markus_schwaninger@med.uni-heidelberg.de

Schwartz, M.
Department of Neurobiology, The Weizmann Institute of Science,
76100 Rehovot, Israel
e-mail: Michal.Schwartz@weizmann.ac.il

Spatz, M.
Stroke Branch, NINDS, NIH, Bldg. 36, Room 4A03,
36 Convent Drive, MSC 4128, Bethesda, MD, 20892-4128, USA
e-mail: Spatzm@ninds.nih.gov

Stock, C.
School of Biological Sciences, University of Manchester,
Oxford Road, Manchester, M13 9PT, UK

Takeda, H.
Stroke Branch, NINDS, NIH, Bldg. 36, Room 4A03,
36 Convent Drive, MSC 4128, Bethesda, MD, 20892-4128, USA
e-mail: icb_th@polka.plala.or.jp

Wolburg, H.
Institute for Pathology, Universität Tübingen, Liebermeisterstr. 8,
72076 Tübingen, Germany
e-mail: hartwig.wolburg@med.uni-tuebingen.de

Wolburg-Buchholz, K.
Max Planck Institute for Vascular Biology, ZMBE,
Von Esmarch-Straße 56, 48149, Münster, Germany

Yrjänheikki, J.
Cerebricon Ltd., Mikrokatu 1, 70210, Kuopio, Finland
e-mail: juha.yrjanheikki@cerebricon.com

del Zoppo, G.J.
Department of Molecular and Experimental Medicine,
The Scripps Research Institute, La Jolla, CA 92037, USA
e-mail: grgdlzop@hermes.scripps.edu

1 Matrix Metalloproteinases in Neuroinflammation and Cerebral Ischemia

G. A. Rosenberg, S. Mun-Bryce

1.1 Introduction

Cerebral ischemia initiates a cascade of molecular events that leads to infarction by necrosis and apoptosis (Ginsberg and Pulsinelli 1994; Dirnagl et al. 1999; Graham and Chen 2000). Neurons and astrocytes are affected early, while blood vessels are more resistant to hypoxia. However, when the vasculature begins to break down, vasogenic edema and hemorrhage result (Klatzo 1967). Since first observed by Fisher and Adams (1951), many investigators have reported that reperfusion increases the damage to the blood–brain barrier (BBB) (Fujimoto et al. 1976; Hallenbeck and Dutka 1990; Yang and Betz 1994; Belayev et al. 1996). Multiple factors contribute to the vascular injury, including the production, release, and activation of proteases. For several years our laboratory has been studying the matrix metalloproteinases (MMPs), a gene family of neutral proteases that degrade all of the components of the extracellular matrix. MMPs are important in normal and pathological changes in the extracellular matrix (Nagase and Woessner 1999). A growing list of neurological diseases have been shown to involve the MMPs. These include multiple sclerosis, bacterial meningitis, cerebral ischemia, Guillian-Barre (blood–nerve barrier), Alzheimer's disease, and HIV dementia (Yong et al. 2001). A major effect of the MMPs is to attack the blood vessels, increasing their permeability and causing breakdown of the BBB (Rosenberg et al. 1992).

Gelatinases (72- and 92-kDa type IV collagenases) attack proteins in the basal lamina and those that form tight junctions between endothelial cells. In neuroinflammation, the gelatinases and other MMPs are produced and activated. We have used an inflammatory response induced by the intracerebral injection of the bacterial cell wall component lipopolysaccharide (LPS) to study the production of proinflammatory MMPs and their relationship to disruption of the BBB. Intracerebral injection of LPS induces gelatinase B (MMP-9) and stromelysin-1 (MMP-3). We have also studied the role of MMPs in disruption of the BBB secondary to cerebral ischemia with reperfusion. In cerebral ischemia, the MMPs appear to be critical in the hemorrhagic transformation that can occur spontaneously and in intracerebral hemorrhage induced by treatment with recombinant tissue plasminogen activator (rt-PA). In ischemia, the timing of the opening is dependent on the length of the ischemic episode, and whether reperfusion occurs.

This review will focus on the role of the MMPs in proteolytic disruption of the BBB in LPS-induced neuroinflammation and in cerebral ischemia. This is important because of the potential to control damage to the BBB with synthetic inhibitors to the MMPs. Several reviews have appeared in the past few years describing the role of the MMP in the central nervous system (Yong et al. 2001; Rosenberg 2002).

1.2 Biology of the Matrix Metalloproteinases

MMPs are classified into four major groups based on the structural elements (Nagase and Woessner 1999). All of the MMPs have a zinc catalytic active site. At the N-terminus, a propeptide blocks the active zinc site. Matrilysin (MMP-7) is the smallest of the MMPs, containing only the propeptide region and zinc catalytic site. Stromelysins (MMP-3 and -10) also have a hemopexin domain. Gelatinases (MMP-2 and -9) have fibronectin binding sites that direct them to the basal lamina, which contains the fibronectin. Some of the family members are attached to the membrane, the membrane-type metalloproteinases (MT-MMP), which are important in the activation of the constitutively produced MMP-2. The latent, inactive state of MMPs is maintained by an unpaired cysteine sulfhydryl group near the C-terminal end that binds with the zinc site. Proteolytic removal or reconfiguration of the cysteine propeptide region activates the MMPs, forming the so-called cysteine switch (Van Wart and Birkedal Hansen 1990).

Gelatinase A is constitutively expressed in the central nervous system, and is found normally in brain tissue and in the cerebrospinal fluid. MMP-2 acts as a housekeeping gene, and the factors involved in its transcription in brain are poorly understood. On the other hand, MMP-9 normally is absent or found at low concentrations. Inflammation results in the marked up-regulation of MMP-9, which is the major MMP found in the inflamed tissues. In contrast to MMP-2, the MMP-9 expression is controlled by a number of transcriptional factors.

Intracerebral injection of MMP-2 results in the opening of the BBB with hemorrhage around the blood vessels. The gelatinase attacks the macromolecules in the basal lamina that surrounds the blood vessels. The main components of the basal lamina are type IV collagen, laminin, fibronectin, and heparan sulfate, all of which are targets of the gelatinases (Rosenberg et al. 1992). MMP-9 was shown to degrade proteins that form the tight junctions between endothelial cells, such as zona occludens-1 and occludins (Harkness et al. 2000). They are also involved in the breakdown of laminin (Hamann et al. 1995). Another important proinflammatory MMP is stromelysin-1 (MMP-3). Microglia and pericytes express MMP-3 in ischemic tissues (Rosenberg et al. 2001).

A new family of metalloproteinases was recently discovered. The *a d*isintegrin *a*nd *m*etalloproteinase (ADAM) gene family of proteases have both metalloproteinase and disintegrin domains (Schlondorff and Blobel 1999). The disintegrin region binds ADAMs to the membrane integrins, and the metalloproteinase domain provides the protease function. This combination makes ADAMs important in events at the cell surface. One of the first ADAMs to be described that had implications in brain function was the tumor-necrosis factor-*a*-converting enzyme or TACE (ADAM-17). TNF-*a* is bound to the membrane as an inactive 26-kDa form, and is processed to an active 17-kDa entity by TACE. Hydroxymate-based metalloproteinase inhibitors block the processing of inactive TNF-*a* to the active form (Gearing et al. 1994; McGeehan et al. 1994). The growing ADAMs family includes enzymes that cleave a number of ECM molecules, acting as "sheddases" to remove ectodomain molecules from the cell surface. Shedding of the TNF-*a* receptor, interleukin-6, L-selectin, and syndecans has been shown to be a function of ADAMs (Yong et al. 2001). ADAMs with a thrombospondin domain (ADAMTS) form another group of metalloproteinases. ADAMTS4 has been shown to degrade aggrecan, and to be involved in spinal cord injury (Lemons et al. 2001).

Plasminogen/plasmin system enzymes interact with the MMPs (Cuzner et al. 1996; Cuzner and Opdenakker 1999). Serine proteases, urokinase-type, and tissue-type plasminogen activators (uPA and tPA, respectively), participate in the activation of the MMPs (Mazzieri et al. 1997; Carmeliet et al. 1997). They are involved in normal extracellular remodeling and angiogenesis, and in the pathological processes associated with tumor growth (Mignatti and Rifkin 1996).

MMPs are secreted in a proform that requires activation. ProMMP-2 is activated by the membrane bound MT-MMP (Sato et al. 1994). Plasmin activates proMMP-3 (Baricos et al. 1995; Nagase 1997). ProMMP-9 is activated by MMP-3 (Ramos-DeSimone et al. 1999). Recent evidence implicates the free radicals, nitric oxide and reactive oxygen species, in the activation of the MMPs. Mice deficient in copper/zinc superoxide dismutase-1 had greater damage to the BBB after ischemia with reperfusion compared to the wild type (Gasche et al. 2001). Nitric oxide activates MMP-9 by a nitroxylation process that appears to involve the propeptide region (Gu et al. 2002).

1.3 Lipopolysaccharide-Induced Neuroinflammation and the Blood–Brain Barrier

Intracerebral injection of cytokines and lipopolysaccharide (LPS) induces an inflammatory response that leads to the opening of the BBB (Wispelwey et al. 1988). LPS injected into the brain is less damaging than in peripheral organs, for reasons that are unclear (Andersson et al. 1992). Earlier, we showed that an intracerebral injection of TNF-a caused the opening of the BBB at 24 h after injection. The opening was related to increased expression of MMP-9. Furthermore, an inhibitor to MMP-9, the hydroxymate-based batimastat (BB-94), blocked the opening, suggesting that the BBB opening was related to the action of a metalloproteinase (Rosenberg et al. 1995).

We have studied the effect of injection of LPS into the caudate nucleus of rats. Assay of MMPs was done by gelatin-substrate zymography in brain tissues at various times after the injection of LPS. LPS produced a significant increase in both latent MMP-9 (92-kDa) with an active species (84-kDa) seen by 4 h (Fig. 1) (Mun-Bryce and Rosenberg 1998). We measured the time-course of the opening of the BBB in the LPS-injected animals, using radiolabeled tracers. Sucrose, a small molecule that remains mainly in the blood, is a sensitive marker of BBB opening. We found that the uptake of sucrose, as measured as a ratio of the levels in the brain to that in the blood was increased, indicating disruption of the BBB (Fig. 2) (Mun-Bryce and Rosenberg 1998). The role of MMPs in the LPS-induced injury to the BBB was further investigated with the use of synthetic MMP inhibitors. Four hours after bilateral LPS or saline intracerebral injection, a group of experimental animals received a 30-mg/kg intraperitoneal injection of the synthetic metalloproteinase inhibitor, BB-1101 (British Biotechnology), which is a broad-spectrum MMP inhibitor that also inhibits ADAM-17 (TACE). BBB permeability was measured 12 h after either LPS or saline injection. Ten minutes before euthanasia, animals received an intravenous dose of [^{14}C]sucrose. Blood and brain tissue samples were collected for liquid scintillation counting. The BB-1101 reduced the BBB opening in the sucrose studies. There was a reduction of the levels of 92- and 84-kDa gelatinase (Fig. 3).

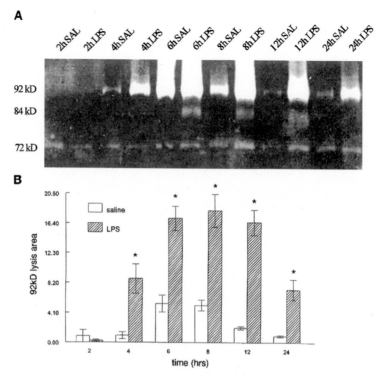

Fig. 1 A, B. Zymography and relative activity values in LPS- vs. saline-injected tissue samples over 24 h. **A** 92- and 84-kDa species of gelatinase B were apparent in zymograms of LPS-stimulated brain tissue samples. The 84-kDa band was absent in saline (SAL)-injected brain tissue samples, whereas activity at the 72-kDa band was unchanged in both experimental groups. **B** Relative activity values of 92-kDa gelatinase B in LPS- vs. saline-injected animals. *Significant differences between saline and LPS ($P<0.01$, $n=4$ tissue samples from the injection site of four animals in each experimental group at each time point). (From Mun-Bryce and Rosenberg 1998)

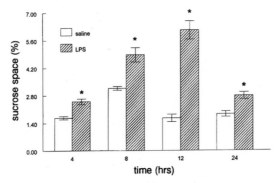

Fig. 2. Brain capillary permeability to [^{14}C]sucrose in LPS- or saline-stimulated brain tissue samples. [^{14}C]Sucrose uptake was significantly elevated in LPS-injected samples at each time point compared to the saline samples. *$P < 0.02$ for [^{14}C]sucrose ($n = 8$ tissue samples from brain hemispheres of four animals in each experimental group at each time point). (From Mun-Bryce and Rosenberg 1998)

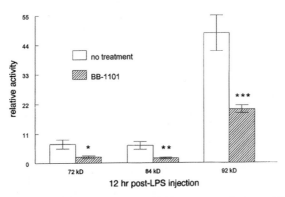

Fig. 3. Intracerebral LPS injection increased 92-kDa gelatinase. Treatment with B-1101 (30 mg/kg) resulted in a decrease in 92- and 84-kDa forms of MMP-9. This fall in MMP-9 corresponded with improvement in BBB permeability seen with BB-1101. (From Mun-Bryce and Rosenberg 1998)

1.4 MMP mRNA and Immunohistochemistry of MMPs After LPS Injection

The effect of the expression of mRNA for the MMPs was studied in LPS-injected animals with a competitive PCR method (Wells et al. 1997). The mRNA of MMP-2 and TNF-α were constitutively expressed in non-injected brain tissue. Two hours following LPS injection, MMP-2 and MMP-3 were significantly up-regulated 30- and 60-fold, respectively, compared to noninjected tissue. MMP-9 and TNF-α mRNA expression was nonsignificantly increased in LPS-injected brain tissue. Saline-injected tissue failed to show a significant rise in any of the observed MMPs or TNF-α at 2 h. The MMPs were increased prior to the expression of the mRNA for the TNF-α (Fig. 4).

The cellular localization of the MMPs was studied 8 h after the injection of LPS, when BBB disruption was maximal. Cryosectioned frozen tissue sections were fixed and immunostained for MMPs. Immunostaining for MMP-2 was absent at the site of LPS-injection as well as in saline-injected brain at 8 h (Mun-Bryce et al. 2002). How-

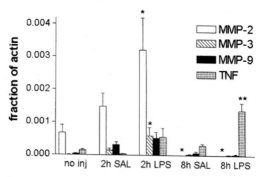

Fig. 4. Semiquantitative PCR of LPS-stimulated tissue. Relative gene expression of MMP-2, -3, and -9, and TNF-α at 2 h and 8 h after LPS or saline injection into the caudate, compared to noninjected controls. MMP-2 and -3 exhibited a marked increase in mRNA expression at 2 h following LPS injection compared to noninjected tissue. Gene expression of MMP-2 and -3 was almost diminished by 8 h, whereas TNF-α mRNA levels showed a 10-fold increase compared to saline-injected and noninjected controls. (From Mun-Bryce et al. 2002)

ever, nearby blood vessels exhibited fine processes of MMP-2 immunoreactivity contacting or projecting to vessels in regions adjacent to the LPS-injected site, in saline-injected brain tissue, and in noninjected tissue of the contralateral hemisphere of LPS-injected brains.

Intense MMP-3 immunoreactivity was evident in cells within and adjacent to the LPS-injection site. In regions near the LPS-injection site, perivascular cells adjacent to blood vessels and in the parenchyma surrounding these vessels contained distinct MMP-3 immunostaining. Similarly but to a lesser degree, MMP-3-positive staining was restricted to cells near the blood vessel interface in saline-injected brains. MMP-3 immunostaining was absent in the cerebrovasculature of the noninjected opposite hemisphere as well as in noninjected control animals. Comparable to the pattern of MMP-3, strong MMP-9 immunoreactivity was detected in and around cells at the LPS injection site and in endothelial and perivascular cells in adjacent blood vessels. Cells with intense MMP-9 immunostaining were localized around the basal lamina layer of these blood vessels. Less intense MMP-9-positive staining was also localized around cerebral vessels in saline-injected tissue. Staining for MMP-9 was absent in noninjected brain tissue from the opposite hemisphere and in noninjected control animals.

In blood vessels adjacent to the LPS injection site, cells immunostaining for the microglia/macrophage marker Ox-42 were observed around the blood vessels. MMP-3 immunostaining cells were found in the same location as the Ox-42^{+} cells. At the injection site, a large number of Ox-42 cells were seen around blood vessels as well as in the surrounding parenchyma. In a similar fashion to Ox-42 staining, MMP-3 was found in a cellular and extracellular pattern. Fluorescent staining with dual labels showed that Ox-42 and MMP-3 were colocalized.

These studies suggest that astrocytes normally secrete MMP-2, which can be activated by the membrane-type MMP, which restricts the proteolysis to the close vicinity of the cell surface. When a more generalized inflammatory response occurs, there is activation of the astrocytes, which release latent MMP-9, and up-regulation of microglia, which release MMP-3. Plasmin may contribute to the process by activation of the MMPs. A schematic drawing of the possible mechanisms of activation of MMP-2 and -9 is shown in Fig. 5.

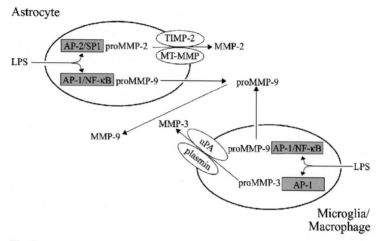

Fig. 5. Astrocytes and microglia secrete and activate the MMPs. Astrocytes form MMP-2 constitutively, and contain membrane-type MMP (*MT-MMP*), which is involved in the activation of the MMP-2. When an inflammatory stimulus is present, the astrocytes make MMP-9. Microglia release MMP-3, which may be activated by the plasmin system, and is an activator of the MMP-9

1.5 MMPs in Neuroinflammation in Cerebral Ischemia

Biochemical studies of MMPs in permanent and temporary ischemia have shown that the gelatinases contribute to the disruption of the BBB that leads to vasogenic cerebral edema and hemorrhage (Mun-Bryce and Rosenberg 1998). Permanent middle cerebral artery occlusion in spontaneously hypertensive rats (SHRs) resulted in the production of MMP-9 by 24 h, and a marked increase in MMP-2 by 5 days (Rosenberg et al. 1996). The increase in MMP-9 correlates with the time of maximal damage, while the later increase in MMP-2 is related to the increase in reactive astrocytes around the cyst. Middle cerebral artery occlusion for 90 min with reperfusion in SHRs caused a biphasic opening of the BBB with a transient opening at 3 h and a second more severe injury at 48 h (Rosenberg et al. 1998). The early opening at 3 h correlated with an increase in MMP-2, while a later opening at the 48 h correlated with increased expression of MMP-9. A hydroxymate MMP inhibitor, BB-1101, blocked the edema at 24 h and the early opening of the BBB at 3 h, but failed to alter the secondary opening of the BBB at 48 h.

MMPs are increased in the mouse stroke model with reperfusion, using a sensitive method of extraction of MMPs from small amounts of tissues (Gasche et al. 1999). A MMP-9 knockout mouse was found to have reduced infarct size and less BBB damage (Asahi et al. 2000, 2001). Hydroxymate MMP inhibitors have been shown to reduce cerebral edema in intracerebral hemorrhage (Rosenberg and Navratil 1997). Thus, there is considerable evidence to support a role for the MMPs in pathological changes associated with cerebral ischemia, particularly with the changes that occur in the cerebral vasculature.

Breakdown of the extracellular matrix proteins that form the basal lamina has been demonstrated by the loss of laminin in infracted tissues in a model of stroke in the nonhuman primate (Hamann et al. 1995). The greater the loss of the laminin, the more likely is hemorrhagic transformation to occur. The levels of MMP-9 are associated with hemorrhagic transformation, while MMP-2 is correlated with neuronal injury (Heo et al. 1999).

Several recent studies have documented a beneficial effect of MMP inhibition in cerebral infarction. Hemorrhagic infarction secondary to multiple emboli infused into the carotid artery of rabbits was reduced with an MMP inhibitor, BB-94 (Lapchak et al. 2000). Prolonged ischemia prior to reperfusion increased the risk of hemorrhages with a high incidence of mortality in the animals with hemorrhages. In a recent study in rodents, BB-94 dramatically reduced mortality (Sumii and Lo 2002). Treatment with BB-94 and rt-PA in rats that had MCAO resulted in the closure of the BBB, preventing the rt-PA from extravasating into the brain, where it is toxic (Pfefferkorn, manuscript submitted).

Human studies have shown the presence of MMPs in the tissues of stroke patients (Clark et al. 1997; Anthony et al. 1997). In patients with stroke, serum levels of MMP-2 and MMP-9 were measured by ELISA in patients with cardioembolic stroke. NIH stroke scores were used to separate the patients into those with severe strokes (NIHSS equal to or greater than 8) and those with milder scores. Those with severe strokes had significantly higher levels of

MMP-9 at baseline, and the elevated levels persisted for 48 h (Montaner et al. 2001 a). When hemorrhagic transformation or parenchymal hemorrhages were present, the highest levels of MMP-9 were found in those patients with late hemorrhagic transformation (Montaner et al. 2001 b).

Studies in a variety of animal species and in humans provide strong evidence that early activation of constituently expressed MMP-2, and up-regulation and activation of proinflammatory MMP-3 and -9 play a major role in the damage to the blood vessels that leads to vasogenic edema and hemorrhage. Most likely, the plasmin/plasminogen system, which activates MT-MMP and MMP-3, plays a role in the process. Free radicals may affect both the activation and induction, but further study will be needed to clarify that role.

Treatment with MMP inhibitors has prevented the BBB damage and reduced the edema in cerebral infarction with reperfusion. Several recent studies have shown that MMP inhibitors are effective in reducing hemorrhage and mortality in animals given recombinant tissue plasminogen activator (rtPA). Current MMP inhibitors are broad-spectrum. Ideally, the primary MMPs involved in the opening of the BBB will be identified and compounds developed to specifically block them. This has been an elusive goal, however. Current MMP inhibitors developed for cancer and arthritis treatment have side effects associated with long-term use. In neurological disorders, short-term use may be possible, avoiding the undesirable side effects.

1.6 Conclusions

Matrix metalloproteinases are involved in the neuroinflammatory response that results in the opening of the BBB and increased risk of hemorrhage. Studies with LPS to induce inflammation have shown an association between the disruption of the BBB and the presence of MMPs. Evidence is emerging that the plasmin/plasminogen system and free radicals interact with the MMPs. Cerebral ischemia leads to over-expression of the MMPs. If the ischemic insult is severe, vasogenic edema and hemorrhage result. The MMPs contribute to hemorrhagic transformation. Synthetic inhibitors of the MMPs block the opening of the BBB, suggesting that they may be used therapeutically to reduce the neuroinflammatory response.

References

Andersson PB, Perry VH, Gordon S (1992) The acute inflammatory response to lipopolysaccharide in CNS parenchyma differs from that in other body tissues. Neurosci 48:169–186

Anthony DC, Ferguson B, Matyzak MK, Miller KM, Esiri MM, Perry VH (1997) Differential matrix metalloproteinase expression in cases of multiple sclerosis and stroke. Neuropath Appl Neurobiol 23(5):406–415

Asahi M, Asahi K, Jung JC, del Zoppo GJ, Fini ME, Lo EH (2000) Role for matrix metalloproteinase 9 after focal cerebral ischemia: effects of gene knockout and enzyme inhibition with BB-94. J Cereb Blood Flow Metab 20(12):1681–1689

Asahi M, Wang X, Mori T, Sumii T, Jung JC, Moskowitz MA et al (2001) Effects of matrix metalloproteinase-9 gene knock-out on the proteolysis of blood-brain barrier and white matter components after cerebral ischemia. J Neurosci 21(19):7724–7732

Baricos WH, Cortez SL, el-Dahr SS, Schnaper HW (1995) ECM degradation by cultured human mesangial cells is mediated by a PA/plasmin/MMP-2 cascade. Kidney Intl 47(4):1039–1047

Belayev L, Busto R, Zhao W, Ginsberg MD (1996) Quantitative evaluation of blood-brain barrier permeability following middle cerebral artery occlusion in rats. Brain Res 739:88–96

Carmeliet P, Moons L, Lijnen R, Baes M, Lemaitre V, Tipping P et al (1997) Urokinase-generated plasmin activates matrix metalloproteinases during aneurysm formation. Nature Genetics 17(4):439–444

Clark AW, Krekoski CA, Bou SS, Chapman KR, Edwards DR (1997) Increased gelatinase A (MMP-2) and gelatinase B (MMP-9) activities in human brain after focal ischemia. Neurosci Lett 238(1–2):53–56

Cuzner ML, Gveric D, Strand C, Loughlin AJ, Paemen L, Opdenakker G (1996) et al. The expression of tissue-type plasminogen activator, matrix metalloproteases and endogenous inhibitor in the central nervous system in multiple sclerosis: Comparison of stages in lesion evolution. J Neuropath Exp Neurol 55:1194–1209

Cuzner ML, Opdenakker G (1999) Plasminogen activators and matrix metalloproteases, mediators of extracellular proteolysis in inflammatory demyelination of the central nervous system. J Neuroimmunol 94(1–2):1–14

Dirnagl U, Iadecola C, Moskowitz MA (1999) Pathobiology of ischaemic stroke: an integrated view. Trends Neurosci 22(9):391–397

Fisher M, Adams RD (1951) Observations on brain embolism with special reference to the mechanism of hemorrhagic infarction. J Exper Neurol Neuropath 10:92–96

Fujimoto T, Walker JT, Spatz M, Klatzo I (1976) Pathophysiologic aspects of ischemic edema. In: Pappius HM, Feindel W (eds). Dynamics of Brain Edema. Springer-Verlag, Berlin, pp 171–180

Gasche Y, Fujimura M, Morita-Fujimura Y, Copin JC, Kawase M, Massengale J (1999) et al. Early appearance of activated matrix metalloproteinase-9 after focal cerebral ischemia in mice: a possible role in blood-brain barrier dysfunction. Journal of Cerebral Blood Flow & Metabolism 19(9):1020–1028

Gasche Y, Copin JC, Sugawara T, Fujimura M, Chan PH (2001) Matrix metalloproteinase inhibition prevents oxidative stress-associated blood-brain barrier disruption after transient focal cerebral ischemia. J Cereb Blood Flow Metab 21(12):1393–1400

Gearing AJ, Beckett P, Christodoulou M, Churchill M, Clements J, Davidson AH (1994) et al. Processing of tumour necrosis factor-alpha precursor by metalloproteinases. Nature 370(6490):555–557

Ginsberg MD, Pulsinelli WA (1994) The ischemic penumbra, injury thresholds, and the therapeutic window for acute stroke. Ann Neurol 36(4):553–554

Graham SH, Chen J (2001) Programmed cell death in cerebral ischemia. J Cereb Blood Flow Metab 21(2):99–109

Gu Z, Kaul M, Yan B, Kridel SJ, Cui J, Strongin A et al (2002) S-nitrosylation of matrix metalloproteinases: signaling pathway to neuronal cell death. Science 297(5584):1186–1190

Hallenbeck JM, Dutka AJ (1990) Background review and current concepts of reperfusion injury. Arch Neurol 47(11):1245–1254

Hamann GF, Okada Y, Fitridge R, del Zoppo GJ (1995) Microvascular basal lamina antigens disappear during cerebral ischemia and reperfusion. Stroke 26(11):2120–2126

Harkness KA, Adamson P, Sussman JD, Davies-Jones GA, Greenwood J, Woodroofe MN (2000) Dexamethasone regulation of matrix metalloproteinase expression in CNS vascular endothelium. Brain 123 (Pt 4):698–709

Heo JH, Lucero J, Abumiya T, Koziol JA, Copeland BR, del Zoppo GJ (1999) Matrix metalloproteinases increase very early during experimental focal cerebral ischemia. J Cereb Blood Fl & Metab 19(6):624–633

Klatzo I (1967) Presidential address. Neuropathological aspects of brain edema. J Neuropathol Exp Neurol 26:1–14

Lapchak PA, Chapman DF, Zivin JA (2000) Metalloproteinase inhibition reduces thrombolytic (tissue plasminogen activator)-induced hemorrhage after thromboembolic stroke. Stroke 31(12):3034–3040

Lemons ML, Sandy JD, Anderson DK, Howland DR (2001) Intact aggrecan and fragments generated by both aggrecans and metalloproteinase-like activities are present in the developing and adult rat spinal cord and their relative abundance is altered by injury. J Neurosci 21(13):4772–4781

Mazzieri R, Masiero L, Zanetta L, Monea S, Onisto M, Garbisa S et al (1997) Control of type IV collagenase activity by components of the urokinase-plasmin system: a regulatory mechanism with cell-bound reactants. EMBO J 16(9):2319–2332

McGeehan GM, Becherer JD, Bast RC Jr., Boyer CM, Champion B, Connolly KM et al (1994) Regulation of tumour necrosis factor-alpha processing by a metalloproteinase inhibitor. Nature 370:558–561

Mignatti P, Rifkin DB (1996) Plasminogen activators and matrix metalloproteinases in angiogenesis. Enzyme & Protein 49(1–3):117–137

Montaner J, Alvarez-Sabin J, Molina C, Angles A, Abilleira S, Arenillas J et al (2001a) Matrix metalloproteinase expression after human cardioembolic stroke: temporal profile and relation to neurological impairment. Stroke 32(8):1759–1766

Montaner J, Alvarez-Sabin J, Molina CA, Angles A, Abilleira S, Arenillas J et al (2001b) Matrix metalloproteinase expression is related to hemorrhagic transformation after cardioembolic stroke. Stroke 32(12):2762–2767

Mun-Bryce S, Rosenberg GA (1998) Gelatinase B modulates selective opening of the blood-brain barrier during inflammation. Am J Physiol 274(5 Pt 2):R1203–11

Mun-Bryce S, Rosenberg GA (1998) Matrix metalloproteinases in cerebrovascular disease. J Cereb Blood Flow & Metab 18(11):1163–1172

Mun-Bryce S, Lukes A, Wallace J, Lukes-Marx M, Rosenberg GA (2002) Stromelysin-1 and gelatinase A are upregulated before TNF-alpha in LPS-stimulated neuroinflammation. Brain Res 933(1):42–49

Nagase H (1997) Activation mechanisms of matrix metalloproteinases. Biol Chem 378(3–4):151–160

Nagase H, Woessner JF, Jr (1999) Matrix metalloproteinases. J Biol Chem 274(31):21491–21494

Ramos-DeSimone N, Hahn-Dantona E, Sipley J, Nagase H, French DL, Quigley et al (1999) Activation of matrix metalloproteinase-9 (MMP-9) via a converging plasmin/stromelysin-1 cascade enhances tumor cell invasion. J Biol Chem 274(19):13066–13076

Rosenberg GA (2002) Matrix metalloproteinases and neuroinflammation in multiple sclerosis. Neurosci 8(6):586–595

Rosenberg GA, Navratil M (1997) Metalloproteinase inhibition blocks edema in intracerebral hemorrhage in the rat. Neurol 48(4):921–926

Rosenberg GA, Kornfeld M, Estrada E, Kelley RO, Liotta LA, Stetler-Stevenson WG (1992) TIMP-2 reduces proteolytic opening of blood-brain barrier by type IV collagenase. Brain Res 576:203–207

Rosenberg GA, Estrada EY, Dencoff JE, Stetler-Stevenson WG (1995) Tumor necrosis factor-alpha-induced gelatinase B causes delayed opening of the blood-brain barrier: an expanded therapeutic window. Brain Res 703:151–155

Rosenberg GA, Navratil M, Barone F, Feuerstein G (1996) Proteolytic cascade enzymes increase in focal cerebral ischemia in rat. J Cereb Blood Flow & Metab 16(3):360–366

Rosenberg GA, Estrada EY, Dencoff JE (1998) Matrix metalloproteinases and TIMPs are associated with blood-brain barrier opening after reperfusion in rat brain. Stroke 29(10):2189–2195

Rosenberg GA, Cunningham LA, Wallace J, Alexander S, Estrada EY, Grossetete M et al (2001) Immunohistochemistry of matrix metalloproteinases in reperfusion injury to rat brain: activation of MMP-9 linked to stromelysin-1 and microglia in cell cultures. Brain Res 893(1–2):104–112

Sato H, Takino T, Okada Y, Cao J, Shinagawa A, Yamamoto E, et al (1994) A matrix metalloproteinase expressed on the surface of invasive tumour cells. Nature 370:61–65

Schlondorff J, Blobel CP (1999) Metalloprotease-disintegrins: modular proteins capable of promoting cell-cell interactions and triggering signals by protein-ectodomain shedding. J Cell Sci 112(Pt 21):3603–3617

Sumii T, Lo EH (2002) Involvement of matrix metalloproteinase in thrombolysis-associated hemorrhagic transformation after embolic focal ischemia in rats. Stroke 33(3):831–836

Van Wart HE, Birkedal Hansen H (1990) The cysteine switch: a principle of regulation of metalloproteinase activity with potential applicability to the entire matrix metalloproteinase gene family. Proc Natl Acad Sci USA 87:5578–5582

Wells GM, Catlin G, Cossins JA, Mangan M, Ward GA, Miller KM et al (1996) Quantitation of matrix metalloproteinases in cultured rat astrocytes using the polymerase chain reaction with a multi-competitor cDNA standard. Glia 18(4):332–340

Wispelwey B, Lesse AJ, Hansen EJ, Scheld WM (1988) Haemophilus influenzae lipopolysaccharide-induced blood brain barrier permeability during experimental meningitis in the rat. J Clin Invest 82:1339–1346

Yang GY, Betz AL (1994) Reperfusion-induced injury to the blood-brain barrier after middle cerebral artery occlusion in rats. Stroke 25(8):1658–64

Yong VW, Power C, Forsyth P, Edwards DR (2001) Metalloproteinases in biology and pathology of the nervous system. Nat Rev Neurosci 2(7):502–511

2 Involvement of Tight Junctions During Transendothelial Migration of Mononuclear Cells in Experimental Autoimmune Encephalomyelitis

H. Wolburg, K. Wolburg-Buchholz, B. Engelhardt

2.1 Introduction

Homeostasis of the neural microenvironment of the central nervous system (CNS) is essential for the normal function of neuronal networks and is protected by the blood–brain barrier (BBB). The BBB is formed by highly specialized capillary endothelial cells, which inhibit transendothelial passage of molecules from blood to brain by an extremely low pinocytotic activity and the lack of fenestrae, and the BBB restricts the paracellular diffusion of hydrophilic molecules due to an elaborate network of complex tight junctions between the endothelial cells. On the other hand, in order to meet the high metabolic requirements of the CNS tissue, specific transport systems are selectively expressed in the capillary brain endothelial cell membranes, which mediate the directed transport of nutrients into the CNS (in particular the glucose transporter) or of toxic metabolites out of the CNS (the multidrug resistance system) (Greenwood et al. 1995).

Because of the presence of the BBB, the lack of lymphatic vessels, and the absence of classical MHC-positive antigen-presenting cells, the CNS has been considered an immunologically privileged site. In fact, under physiological conditions, lymphocyte entry into the healthy CNS is kept at a low level (Wekerle et al. 1986). However, during inflammatory diseases of the CNS, circulating immunocompetent cells get access to the CNS. The understanding of the stimulation and infiltration into the brain of inflammatory cells, the consecutive activation of microglia and astrocytes, and their upregulated release of a number of different cytokines which are directed against many partners of this immense network of cellular reactions is still at its beginning (Weiner and Selkoe 2002).

The endothelial cell barrier is directly located at the interface between blood and brain and must be crossed by inflammatory cells. Therefore, the molecular changes at the BBB during CNS inflammation are in the focus of interest. They lead to loss of barrier properties and subsequently to edema formation, exacerbation of disease, and chronic inflammatory cell recruitment into the CNS, which are critically involved in the pathogenesis of multiple sclerosis (MS) and experimental autoimmune encephalomyelitis (EAE) (Stanimirovic and Satoh 2000). The role of tight junctions in the process of transendothelial migration of inflammatory cells across the BBB is not yet understood. Most investigators prefer the model of a paracellular route of transendothelial migration of mononuclear cells by compromising tight junctions (for a recent example, see Mamdouh et al. 2003), but there are other known mechanisms of how leukocytes can cross the endothelial barrier (Feng et al. 2002). On the other hand, tight junction molecules can be lost from endothelial cell-cell contacts during CNS inflammation, suggesting their possible involvement in the process of inflammatory cell recruitment. However, the relation between change in tight junction protein expression and the tight junction-independent leukocyte transmigration is not yet understood.

2.2 Morphology of the BBB

In the brain parenchyma, the BBB is located in the endothelial cells and restricts the paracellular diffusion of hydrophilic molecules by both complex tight junctions (Reese and Karnovsky 1967; Brightman and Reese 1969) and a low number of pinocytotic vesicles as the morphological correlate of transcytosis (Peters et al. 1991). This implies the necessity of various specific transporters for providing the brain with compounds essential for the brain energy metabolism. In brain areas such as in the hypothalamus-neurohypophyseal system, where neurosecretory cells release their neurohormones into the circulation, the blood vessels must be leaky. To avoid a free access of blood-borne substances from these fenestrated vessels to the cerebrospinal fluid (CSF) in the brain ventricle, these brain areas including the circumventricular organs are protected by the blood–CSF barrier. This barrier is complementary to the BBB and is located in the tanycytes of the circumventricular organs, which are glial cells related to ependymal cells. As well, in the choroid plexus, which is the site of CSF production from the blood, the choroid plexus endothelial cells are fenestrated and the blood–CSF barrier is located within the plexus epithelial cells. Again, plexus epithelial cells are related to ependymal cells, and the blood–CSF barrier itself is structurally connected to tight junctions as in the endothelial BBB.

Endothelial and epithelial cells are based by a basal lamina consisting of a large number of molecules of the extracellular matrix. In the endothelial BBB, pericytes and astrocytes are located beyond the basal lamina (Fig. 1). Pericytes are completely surrounded by a basal lamina, whereas the astrocytes contact the basal lamina only with their end-feet. In precapillary arterioles and postcapillary venules, there is commonly a large perivascular space between the endothelium including their associated pericytes or smooth muscle cells and the glial limiting membrane. Thus, in contrast to the BBB, where a common basal lamina connects endothelial cells with the glial end-feet, pre- and postcapillary vascular profiles have two distinct basal laminae, the vascular one and the glial one (Fig. 2).

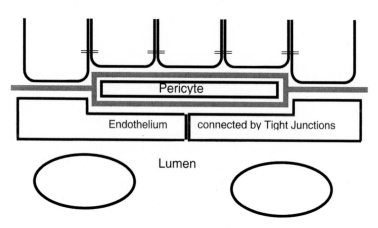

Fig. 1. Highly schematic view of the topology of a blood–brain barrier (BBB) capillary. The endothelial and glial basal lamina are fused together. The pericyte is completely surrounded by a basal lamina. The astrocytic end-feet contact the glial basal lamina and are connected by gap junctions

2.2.1 The Perivascular Microenvironment

The perivascular microenvironment consists of pericytes, astrocytes, and the extracellular matrix.

Pericytes are found in close association with endothelial cells, even at very early stages of development, and seem to be more prevalent on neural capillaries than on other capillaries (Balabanov and Dore-Duffy 1998). Thus, they seem to be necessary for vessel stabilization (Sims 1986). Absence of pericytes as observed after deletion of the gene for the platelet-derived growth factor (PDGF) resulted in hemorrhages (Lindahl et al. 1997). Early during embryogenesis, pericytes are involved in endothelial-neuroectodermal interactions inducing a "commitment" in endothelial cells to form a BBB. This has been documented in the developing chicken CNS, where angiogenic vessels invading the neuroectoderm express *N*-cadherin between endothelial cells and pericytes. With the onset of barrier differentiation, *N*-cadherin labeling decreased, suggesting that transient

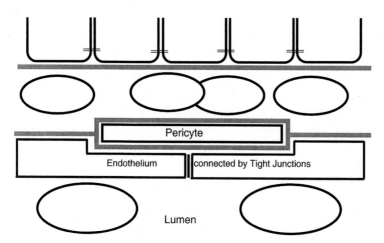

Fig. 2. Highly schematic view of the topology of a postcapillary venule, where the endothelial and glial basal laminae are separated from each other. During inflammation, the leukocytes must penetrate the endothelial basal lamina to reach the perivascular space, and further the glial basal lamina to reach the neural parenchymal compartment

N-cadherin expression in endothelial and perivascular cells may represent an initial signal which may be involved in the commitment of early blood vessels to express BBB properties (Gerhardt et al. 1999). Interestingly, in human glioma blood vessels, we were able to observe an upregulation of *N*-cadherin (Rascher-Eggstein and Wolburg, in preparation), which is obviously reminiscent of early developmental stages of chicken brain microvessels (Gerhardt et al. 1999).

Concerning the other perivascular cell type, the astrocyte, it is generally accepted now that they play a decisive role in the maintenance if not induction of the BBB (Janzer and Raff 1987; for an overview, see Kniesel and Wolburg 2000). Unfortunately, as of this writing nothing is known about which molecules are involved in this induction process. In the mature and normal brain, the astroglial membranes are characterized by the occurrence of orthogonal arrays of particles (OAPs) with a high density where the glial cells contact the basal lamina at the surface of the brain and around blood vessels. In contrast, within the neuropil, the astroglial membranes express only a few OAPs. This polarity of astrocytes, which arises concomitantly with the maturation of the BBB, is not maintained by cultured astrocytes (Wolburg 1995; Nico et al. 2001) and decreases under tumor conditions (Neuhaus 1990). The OAPs were described to contain at least the water channel-forming protein aquaporin-4 (AQP4; for a review, see Venero et al. 2001). The role of OAP/AQP4 in the water homeostasis of the brain and the maintenance of the BBB has been shown by different approaches (Manley et al. 2000; Frigeri et al. 2001; Ke et al. 2001). Furthermore, the development of the OAP/AQP4-related polarity of astrocytes seems to correlate with the time schedule of agrin expression. Agrin, a heparan sulfate proteoglycan, was first isolated from the electric organ of *Torpedo californica* and reported to be essential for clustering acetylcholine receptors in the postsynaptic membrane of the motor endplate (McMahan 1990). Agrin accumulates in the brain microvascular basal lamina during development of the BBB (Barber and Lieth 1997). Since agrin is linked to the cytoskeleton via dystroglycan and the dystrophin-glycoprotein complex (Blake and Kröger 2000), it could participate in establishing a cellular polarity, which is a characteristic feature of perivascular astrocytes. In any case, the extracellular matrix of leaky blood vessels in malignant human brain tumors in which barrier-related tight junction molecules were dysregulated was found to be devoid of agrin (Rascher et al. 2002).

2.2.2 Tight Junctions of the BBB

The endothelial cells of the BBB have been shown to form the most complex tight junction networks among all endothelial cells of the whole vasculature of the body (Nagy et al. 1984). The complexity of the network of tight junction strands has been used for the prediction of the physiological parameters permeability and transepithelial electrical resistance (Claude 1978; Claude and Goodenough 1973, Marcial et al. 1984). Although this relationship between morphological and physiological parameters was originally established for epithelial cells, its validity for endothelial cells was also confirmed on the basis of Claude's paradigm. In addition to the network complexity, another morphological parameter of the barrier quality has been established, the association of the tight junction particles with the inner (P-face) or outer (E-face) leaflet of the membrane. In the BBB endothelial cell, the association of tight junction strands with the P-face is approximately as high as that with the E-face. This is in sharp contrast to endothelial cell tight junctions of peripheral blood vessels, which are nearly completely associated with the E-face. Interestingly, the freeze-fracture morphology of tight junctions of peripheral endothelial cells in vivo strongly resembles that of BBB endothelial cells in vitro (Wolburg et al. 1994). This, together with the observation that the BBB-related distribution of tight junction particles is developmentally regulated (Kniesel et al. 1996), gives rise to two important suggestions: (1) the attachment of the tight junction particles with the one or the other membrane leaflet determines the BBB permeability, and (2) the low BBB permeability is not a feature of brain capillary endothelial cells per se, but rather is the result of the interaction of endothelial cells with the brain microenvironment.

The molecular composition of tight junctions is not yet completely known. In recent years, several proteins were identified which are associated with epithelial and endothelial tight junctions. Tight junction-associated proteins include cytoplasmic peripheral membrane proteins of the membrane-associated guanylate kinase (MAGUK) family such as ZO-1, ZO-2, and ZO-3 (reviewed by Tsukita et al. 1999). Integral membrane proteins exclusively localized at tight junctions are occludin and the claudins, which comprise a novel gene-family of four-transmembrane tight junction proteins with no sequence homology to occludin (Furuse et al. 1998a, Morita et al. 1999b). Mice carrying a null mutation in the occludin gene develop morphologically normal tight junctions in most tissues including the brain (Saitou et al. 2000), proving that occludin is not essential for proper tight junction formation. In contrast, transfection of claudins into fibroblasts induced tight junctions in the absence of occludin demonstrating that claudins are essential for tight junction induction. To date, 20 members of the claudin family with different tissue distribution have been described (Mitic et al. 2000). In the CNS, claudin-1, claudin-3, and claudin-5 have been detected in BBB endothelium at the protein level (Liebner et al. 2000a; Morita et al. 1999a); however, only claudin-3 and claudin-5 seem to be incorporated into tight junction strands (Wolburg et al. 2003).

Functional investigations support the view that the composition of the claudin species directly determines permeability parameters of epi- and endothelial cells (Furuse et al. 2001). When transfected in tight junction-negative L-fibroblasts, claudin-1 and claudin-3 form tight junctions associated with the P-face (Furuse et al. 1999). When transfected with claudin-2 or claudin-5, the cells form tight junctions associated with the E-face (Furuse et al. 1998b; Morita et al. 1999a). Together with the morphological observations described above, these transfection experiments suggest that the association of tight junction particles with the membrane leaflets correlates with the stoichiometry of the proteins in a given tight junction. Claudin-3 may contribute to the P-face association, and claudin-5 may contribute to the E-face association in BBB tight junctions (Liebner et al. 2000a; Wolburg et al. 2003). Under pathological conditions, for example in a brain tumor, claudin-3 is lost (Wolburg et al. 2003), together with the P-face-associated particles (Liebner et al. 2000b). In addition, other mechanisms of modulating the attachment of the tight junction proteins with the cytoskeleton may contribute to barrier alterations, as observed in stroke-prone spontaneously hypertensive rats, in which the immunoreactivity of tight junction proteins was unchanged in the BBB, but the E-face association of the brain endothelial cell tight junctions increased (Lippoldt et al. 2000).

2.3 The BBB in the Inflamed Brain

Disruption of the BBB during CNS inflammation can lead to immediate problems of vasogenic edema and the clinical problems related to this condition. Indeed, vascular changes in MS and EAE are pronounced. Active lesions are characterized by the perivascular accumulation of serum components such as albumin or fibrin and inflammatory cells. Whereas the accumulation of serum components in the perivascular space of CNS microvessels demonstrates that passive diffusion of these proteins occurs across the BBB at the same time, the absence of neutrophils and red blood cells within the CNS suggests that even the impaired BBB still plays an active role in the recruitment of inflammatory cells into the CNS. In EAE, leakiness of the BBB occurs mainly at the level of postcapillary venules, which are surrounded by inflammatory cuffs (Fig. 2). CNS postcapillary venules are thin-walled and mainly comprised of endothelial cells, and function as exchange microvessels, much like capillaries (Fenstermacher et al. 2001). Several observations suggest that these small venules are the microvessels that are most prone to disruption and BBB breakdown.

2.3.1 Leukocyte Transmigration

In general, lymphocyte recruitment across the vascular wall is regulated by the sequential interaction of different adhesion or signaling molecules on lymphocytes and endothelial cells lining the vessel wall (Butcher et al. 1999). An initial transient contact of the circulating leukocyte with the vascular endothelium, generally mediated by adhesion molecules of the selectin family and their respective carbohydrate ligands, slows down the leukocyte in the bloodstream (Vestweber 2000). Subsequently, the leukocyte rolls along the vascular wall with greatly reduced velocity. The rolling leukocyte can receive endothelial signals, resulting in its firm adhesion to the endothelial surface. These signals are transduced by chemokines via G-protein-coupled receptors on the leukocyte surface. Binding of a chemokine to its receptor results in a pertussis toxin-sensitive activation of integrins on the leukocyte surface. Only activated integrins mediate the firm adhesion of the leukocytes to the vascular endothelium by binding to their endothelial ligands, which belong to the immunoglobulin (Ig) superfamily. This ultimately leads to the extravasation of the leukocyte. Successful recruitment of circulating leukocytes into the tissue depends on the productive leukocyte/endothelial interaction during each of these sequential steps.

We and others have investigated the expression of adhesion molecules on CNS endothelium during EAE in the SJL/N mouse by means of in situ hybridization and immunohistology and found induction of ICAM-1 and VCAM-1 but not E- and P-selectin on CNS endothelium (Engelhardt et al. 1997; Cannella et al. 1991; Steffen et al. 1994). ICAM-1 and VCAM-1 were shown to mediate adhesion of lymphocytes to inflamed cerebral vessels on frozen brain sections in vitro (Steffen et al. 1994). In vivo monoclonal antibody inhibition studies confirmed the involvement of VCAM-1 and its ligand α4-integrin in the pathogenesis of EAE, as antibodies directed against VCAM-1 and its ligand α4-integrin successfully blocked the development of clinical EAE in the SJL/N mouse. Antibodies against E- and P-selectin did not block EAE development (Engelhardt et al. 1997, 1998).

By applying a novel technique of intravital fluorescence microscopy that allows us to visualize the interaction of circulating encephalitogenic T-lymphoblasts within the healthy spinal cord white matter microvasculature in vivo, we demonstrated that lymphocyte recruitment across microvessels is unique due to the lack of rolling. Constitutively expressed VCAM-1 mediates the G-protein-independent prompt arrest (capture) of circulating encephalitogenic T-cell blasts via α4-integrin to the endothelium of the healthy BBB. Transient capture was followed by G-protein-dependent α4-integrin/ VCAM-1-mediated adhesion strengthening and subsequent leukocyte function antigen-1 (LFA-1)-mediated migration of lymphocytes across the BBB into the spinal cord white matter (Vajkoczy et al. 2001; Laschinger et al. 2002). The requirement for α4-integrin in leukocyte interaction with the inflamed BBB during ongoing EAE is maintained, as demonstrated by intravital microscopy of CNS microvessels in the brain (Kerfoot and Kubes 2002). Furthermore, as recently demonstrated, the requirement for α4-integrin in inflammatory cell recruitment across the BBB seems to translate to the mechanisms involved in inflammatory cell recruitment across the BBB in MS, where therapy using a humanized anti-α4-integrin antibody has proven to be beneficial (von Andrian and Engelhardt 2003).

Morphological analysis of mononuclear recruitment gives no information on the molecular scenario which is initiated at the endothelial cell and within the perivascular space, but it is able to visualize directly the dynamics of structural alterations, which are a challenge for molecular investigations. During EAE, we see a dramatic alteration of the endothelial cell morphology which is characterized by two main features: (1) the consistent maintenance of endothelial

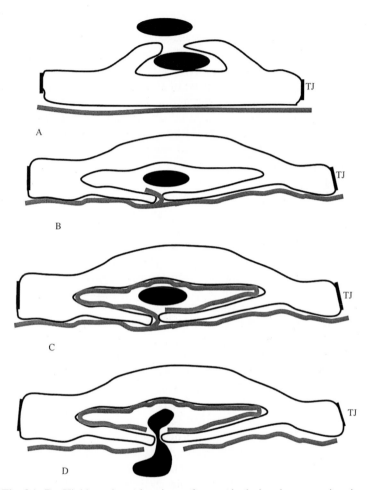

Fig. 3 A–D. Highly schematic view of emperipolesis, the transmigration mode without direct involvement of interendothelial junctions. **A** In a first step, the endothelial cell is induced to fold the luminal membrane, giving rise to a sluice-like chamber. **B** The transformation of a formerly luminal membrane to a novel abluminal membrane. **C** The release of new extracellular matrix at membranes which were formerly directed at the vessel lumen. **D** Finally, a captured leukocyte moves through the abluminal clefts of the endothelial cell by dissolving the basal lamina. *TJ*, tight junction

tight junctions, and (2) the formation of endothelial cavities (Fig. 3). The cavity is established by a dichotomy of the endothelial cell forming a luminal and an abluminal process, leading to a sluice-like chamber (Fig. 3 A). This has been described as occurring during transendothelial transmigration without involvement of intercellular junctions (emperipolesis) (Åström et al. 1968; Rapoport 1976). During emperipolesis, the luminal membrane is folded, forming abluminally directed domains of the sluice chamber. Later on, when the abluminal portion of the chamber opens to give access to the subendothelial space (Fig. 3 B), the former luminal membrane requires a basal lamina, thus definitively defining a novel abluminal membrane (Fig. 3 C, D). This morphological observation is far from being understood in molecular terms. Membrane domains of the endothelial cell must be recommitted by releasing components of the extracellular matrix through membranes which formerly have been directed to the vascular lumen. Through these alterations of the endothelial polarity, the directionality of mononuclear cell transmigration may be influenced in an unknown way, possibly by reorganization of the pattern of adhesion molecules.

Mamdouh et al. (2003) reported on a subjunctional reticulum of PECAM-bearing membranes in cultured human umbilical vein endothelial cells (HUVECs) involved in the redistribution and recycling of surface-connected compartments during transmigration of monocytes. This reticulum apparently was continuous with the surface domains at the intercellular border where PECAM molecules were inserted and involved in homophilic interaction with PECAM on the monocytes. Thus, under the experimental conditions described, PECAM-bearing membrane domains are involved in targeted membrane delivery. However, these PECAM-positive domains were not shown to be junctional domains, because no tight junctional molecules were detected or colocalized. In addition, in our in vivo material, we never found an accumulation of vesicles or other membranes reminiscent of a "subjunctional reticulum" near the tight junctions of brain microvessels revealing monocyte transmigration, but this was the case in in vitro investigations using brain capillary endothelial cells in coculture with astrocytes (Hamm et al., submitted). Thus, the role of surface-connected membrane domains in leukocyte transmigration in HUVECs probably cannot be compared with a processes of transendothelial migration of monocytes across cerebral postcapillary venules during EAE.

2.3.2 Involvement of the BBB Basal Lamina in EAE

A critical step in CNS inflammation is the extravasation of leukocytes from the bloodstream into the CNS parenchyma, which involves autoaggressive T-cell adhesion to and migration through the endothelial cell monolayer of the postcapillary venules. However, after passage across the endothelial cell monolayer, leukocytes still face the endothelial basal lamina, and the subjacent glia limitans consisting of astrocyte end-feet and associated glial basal lamina.

Ultrastructurally, at least two basal laminae can be identified in association with larger blood vessels in the brain, an endothelial one and an astroglial one (Fig. 2). Collectively, both the superficial and the perivascular glial-limiting membranes delineate the border to the brain parenchyma. The endothelial and glial basal laminae define the inner and outer limits of the perivascular space where leukocytes accumulate during acute EAE before infiltrating the brain parenchyma. However, studies to date have not distinguished between penetration of the endothelial cell basement membrane and the process of parenchymal invasion across the glia limitans. There is evidence which suggests that these two steps are distinct and independent of one another: In EAE induced in macrophage-depleted mice (Tran et al. 1998) or in TNF$^{-/-}$ mice (Körner et al. 1997), the inflammatory infiltrate becomes entrapped in the perivascular space and parenchymal infiltration is prevented, indicating that progression through the astrocyte basement membrane is functionally distinct from endothelial cell basement membrane transmigration.

The use of encephalitogenic T-cell lines in in vitro adhesion assays has permitted definition of cell-matrix interactions permissive or restrictive for T-cell extravasation. It has been shown that endothelial cell basement membranes containing laminin 8 are permissive for T-cell transmigration, while those containing laminin 10 are restrictive for T-cell transmigration. Penetration of the parenchymal basement membrane, characterized by the expression of laminins 1 and 2, which are not adhesive for T-cells, occurs only after disruption of this outer barrier, probably via proteolysis and involving matrix metalloproteinases (MMPs) (Graesser et al. 2000; Sixt et al. 2001).

MMPs have been demonstrated to be involved in T-cell entry into and residency in the parenchyma of the CNS, as well as in demyelination. While protease inhibitors have been shown to reduce the severity or delay the onset of EAE, they have not been shown to completely ablate T-cell migration into the perivascular space or the brain parenchyma (Graesser et al. 2000). The results of the MMP inhibitor experiments were, therefore, interpreted as reduced transmigration across the endothelial basal lamina. However, they can equally well be explained by inhibition of transmigration across the glial basal lamina. It now remains to define the main targets of MMP activity, whether they are components of the endothelial or the glial basal lamina.

Distribution of the major laminin receptors, integrin $\alpha6\beta1$ and α-dystroglycan, demonstrated that $\alpha6\beta1$ occurs predominantly on the endothelial cells in the brain mediating interactions with the endothelial cell laminins 8 and 10, while α-dystroglycan is expressed on the astrocyte end-feet and probably mediates binding to the parenchymal laminins 1 and 2 as well as agrin. It has been shown that during the course of EAE, integrin $\alpha6\beta1$ is downregulated on the endothelial cells at sites of infiltration (Sobel et al. 1998). This in combination with our observed high turnover of laminin $\alpha4$ in endothelial cell basement membrane in the brain and the selective upregulation of laminin $\alpha4$ expression by cytokines such as TNF-α which have been shown to play a role in EAE, may lead to a loosening of the endothelial cell-basal lamina interaction, resulting in the reported "rounding up" of endothelial cells observed at sites of T-cell infiltration in EAE (Wolburg et al. 1999), further facilitating the infiltration process.

No information is available about the expression level of endothelial agrin in EAE. As discussed above, agrin is believed to have a benefit for the induction and maintenance of the BBB and is lost in human glioma vessels. Probably, the loss of agrin as reported in glioma blood vessels (Rascher et al. 2002) is causative for the loss of orthogonal arrays of particles (OAP-)/aquaporin-4-related polarity (Neuhaus 1990) in these glioma cells by the reduction if not deletion of the agrin-α-dystroglycan binding activity at the astroglial end-foot membrane. The loss of agrin in turn has been shown to correlate with the loss of tight junctions in the BBB endothelial cells (Rascher et al. 2002). However, the distribution of agrin in the endothelial versus glial basal laminae in postcapillary venules and the reaction of astroglial end-foot-associated molecules such as members of the dystrophin-dystroglycan complex to the EAE-related leukocyte transmigration have not yet been investigated.

2.3.3 Modulation of BBB Tight Junctions in EAE

It is a striking and consistent observation that vessel profiles surrounded by a cuff of transmigrated mononuclear cells are characterized not only by an increase of the luminal surface as described above, but by a complicated and branched course of the tight junctional domains as well. This electron microscopy observation has its immunocytochemical counterpart in the seemingly disrupted tight junction protein-related immunoreactive structures (Plumb et al. 2002) which, in normal BBB, consist of straight and continuous patterns. If the tight junctions develop a complicated three-dimensional scaffold of junctional membranes, the pattern of immunoreactive junctional proteins must appear as discontinuous in the plane of the two-dimensional section.

Using conventional electron microscopy ultrathin sections of postcapillary venules of brains derived from SJL/N mice afflicted with active EAE, we did not observe a direct opening of endothelial tight junctions. We followed mononuclear cell processes through serial ultrathin sections and found the transmigration site apart from the location of tight junctions. This observation completely agrees with the work of the Dvorak group published during the past few years (as summarized in Feng et al. 2002). As well, the observation of intact tight junctions near hemorrhagic interruptions of blood vessels in mice with targeted gene deletions (Sato et al. 1995) supports the view that endothelial tight junctions are considerably stable connections which do not open during transmigration events of different cause.

However, using immunohistochemistry we recently demonstrated that during the clinical disease of EAE, the tight junction molecule claudin-3 is selectively lost from vessels surrounded by inflammatory cuffs (Wolburg et al. 2003). In contrast to claudin-3, the presence of other tight junction molecules such as claudin-5, occludin, or ZO-1 in cerebral vessels was not affected during EAE. These observations differ from a previous report where loss of ZO-1 and occludin from cerebral vascular endothelium was observed during CNS inflammation caused by injection of LPS in juvenile rats (Bolton et al. 1998). However, in that study the cellular infiltrate was dominated by neutrophils, which is in contrast to EAE, where the cellular infiltrate is mostly composed of mononuclear cells. Interestingly, only juvenile rats younger than 3 weeks old developed LPS-induced neutrophil-mediated inflammation in the CNS, whereas injection of LPS in older rats did not lead to any CNS inflammation or alterations at the BBB, indicating that maturation of the BBB was not complete at that age. Thus, loss of occludin and ZO-1 from cerebral vessels upon neutrophil recruitment might be specific to the immature BBB of juvenile rats. Alternatively, recruitment of different leukocyte populations might cause different alterations of the tight junctions due to usage of different routes of transendothelial migration, i.e., transcellular versus paracellular through the tight junctions (Faustmann and Dermietzel 1985; Greenwood et al. 1994). Interestingly, selective loss of claudin-3 can also be observed in leaky vessels in glioblastoma multiforme in the absence of any inflammation, suggesting that in vivo the loss of claudin-3 from BBB tight junctions correlates with BBB breakdown at these sites and that this is not necessarily dependent on the presence of inflammatory cells (Wolburg et al. 2003). Claudin-3 might therefore be a key component determining the permeability of BBB endothelial tight junctions in vivo.

Taken together, we have seen that the morphological stability of endothelial tight junctions does not rule out molecular alterations such as the loss of at least claudin-3 from the tight junctions. In our electron microscopy investigation of EAE material, we found fibrin and electron-dense proteins in the edematously swollen subendothelial space around inflammatory cells, indicating leakage through the inflamed vessel wall. Keeping in mind closed but molecularly altered tight junctions, this could mean that the tight junctions represent a type of molecular sieve not allowing penetration of cells but filtering molecules by their molecular size. Obviously, serum proteins could invade the perivascular space from the vessel lumen, although the number of caveolae or pinocytotic vesicles had not been apparently increased.

2.4 Conclusions

The endothelial cells of the BBB are involved in the pathogenesis of inflammatory demyelinating diseases such as MS or its animal model EAE. Contribution of the BBB can be considered twofold, an active role by guiding inflammatory cells across the BBB and a passive role characterized by breakdown of the BBB.

It has been more than 100 years since the discovery of the BBB. During the last 10 years great progress has been made in understanding the active contribution of the BBB by characterization of the traffic signals involved in leukocyte recruitment into the CNS. However, a uniform mechanism of how the traffic itself is executed, whether the leukocytes travel through the cells or between the cells or both, is not generally accepted yet. In addition, the molecular mechanisms related to the interaction between leukocyte transmigration and compromising tight junctions leading to BBB breakdown are even less understood.

For this purpose, it will be mandatory to characterize the mechanisms involved in BBB differentiation during development and those involved in maintaining BBB characteristics in endothelial cells in the adult CNS.

References

Åström KE, Webster HD, Arnason BG (1968) The initial lesion in experimental allergic neuritis. A phase and electron microscopic study. J Exp Med 128:469–495

Balabanov R, Dore-Duffy P (1998) Role of the CNS microvascular pericyte in the blood-brain barrier. J Neurosci Res 53:637–644

Barber AJ, Lieth E (1997) Agrin accumulates in the brain microvascular basal lamina during development of the blood-brain barrier. Develop Dyn 208:62–74

Blake DJ, Kröger S (2000) The neurobiology of Duchenne muscular dystrophy: learning lessons from muscle? Trends Neurosci 2:92–99

Bolton SJ, Anthony DC, Perry VH (1998) Loss of tight junction proteins occludin and zonula occludens-1 from cerebral vascular endothelium during neutrophil-induced blood-brain barrier breakdown in vivo. Neurosci 86:1245–1257

Brightman MW, Reese TS (1969) Junctions between intimately apposed cell membranes in the vertebrate brain. J Cell Biol 40:648–677

Butcher EC, Williams M, Youngman K, Rott L, Briskin M (1999) Lymphocyte trafficking and regional immunity. Adv Immunol 72:209–253

Cannella B, Cross AH, Raine CS (1991) Adhesion-related molecules in the central nervous system. Upregulation correlates with inflammatory cell influx during relapsing experimental autoimmune encephalomyelitis. Lab Invest 65:23–31

Claude P (1978) Morphologic factors influencing transepithelial permeability. A model for the resistance of the zonula occludens. J Membrane Biol 39:219–232

Claude P, Goodenough DA (1973) Fracture faces of zonulae occludentes from "tight" and "leaky" epithelia. J Cell Biol 58:390–400

Engelhardt B, Vestweber D, Hallmann R, Schulz M (1997) E- and P-selectin are not involved in the recruitment of inflammatory cells across the blood-brain barrier in experimental autoimmune encephalomyelitis. Blood 90: 4459–4472

Engelhardt B, Laschinger M, Schulz M, Samulowitz U, Vestweber D, Hoch G (1998) The development of experimental autoimmune encephalomyelitis in the mouse requires alpha4-integrin but not alpha4beta7-integrin. J Clin Invest 102:2096–2105

Faustmann PM, Dermietzel R (1985) Extravasation of polymorphonuclear leukocytes from the cerebral microvasculature. Cell Tissue Res 242:399–407

Feng D, Nagy JA, Dvorak HF, Dvorak AM (2002) Ultrastructural studies define soluble macromolecular, particulate, and cellular transendothelial cell pathways in venules, lymphatic vessels, and tumor-associated microvessels in man and animals. Micr Res Techn 57:289–326

Fenstermacher J D, Nagaraja T, Davies KR (2001) Overview of the structure and function of the blood-brain barrier in vivo. In: Blood-Brain Barrier: Drug delivery and brain pathology, D Kobiler, S Lustig, S Shapira, eds (New York, Kluwer Academic Plenum Publishers), pp. 1–7

Frigeri A, Nicchia GP, Nico B, Quondamatteo F, Herken R, Roncali L, Svelto M (2001) Aquaporin-4 deficiency in skeletal muscle and brain of dystrophic mdx mice. FASEB J 15: 90–98

Furuse M, Fujita K, Hiiragi T, Fujimoto K, Tsukita S (1998 a) Claudin-1 and -2: novel integral membrane proteins localizing at tight junctions with no sequence similarity to occludin. J Cell Biol 141:1539–1550

Furuse M, Sasaki H, Fujimoto K, Tsukita S (1998 b) A single gene product, claudin-1 or -2, reconstitutes tight junction strands and recruits occludin in fibroblasts. J Cell Biol 143:391–401

Furuse M, Furuse K, Sasaki H, Tsukita S (2001) Conversion of Zonulae occludentes from tight to leaky strand type by introducing claudin-2 into Madin-Darby canine kidney I cells. J Cell Biol 153:263–272

Furuse M, Sasaki H, Tsukita S (1999) Manner of interaction of heterogeneous claudin species within and between tight junction strands. J Cell Biol 147:891–903

Gerhardt H, Liebner S, Redies C, Wolburg H (1999) N-cadherin expression in endothelial cells during early angiogenesis in the eye and brain of the chicken: relation to blood-retina/blood-brain barrier development. Europ J Neurosci 11:1191–1201

Graesser D, Mahooti S, Madri JA (2000) Distinct roles for metalloproteinase-2 and α4 integrin in autoimmune T cell extravasation and residency in brain parenchyma during experimental autoimmune encephalomyelitis. J Neuroimmunol 109:121–131

Greenwood J, Begley DJ, Segal MB (1995) New concepts of blood-brain barrier. Plenum Press, New York, London

Greenwood J, Howes R, Lightman S (1994) The blood-retinal barrier in experimental autoimmune uveoretinitis–leukocyte interactions and functional damage. Lab Invest 70:39–52

Janzer RC, Raff MC (1987) Astrocytes induce blood-brain barrier properties in endothelial cells. Nature 325: 253–257

Ke C, Poon WS, Ng HK, Pang JCS, Chan Y (2001) Heterogenous responses of aquaporin-4 in oedema formation in a replicated severe traumatic brain injury model in rats. Neurosci Letters 301:21–24

Kerfoot S, Kubes P (2002) Overlapping roles of P-selectin and alpha 4 integrin to recruit leukocytes to the central nervous system in experimental autoimmune encephalomyelitis. J Immunol 169:1000–1006

Kniesel U, Risau W, Wolburg H (1996) Development of blood-brain barrier tight junctions in the rat cortex. Dev Brain Res 96:229–240

Kniesel U, Wolburg H (2000) Tight junctions of the blood-brain barrier. Cell Mol Neurobiol 20:57–76

Körner H, Riminton DS, Strickland DH, Lemckert FA, Pollard JD, Sedgwick JD (1997) Critical points of tumor necrosis factor action in central nervous system autoimmune inflammation defined by gene targeting. J Exp Med 186:1585–1590

Laschinger M, Vajkoczy P, Engelhardt B (2002) LFA-1 is not involved in G-protein dependent adhesion of encephalitogenic T cell blasts to CNS microvessels in vivo. Eur J Immmunol 32:3598–3606

Liebner S, Kniesel U, Kalbacher H, Wolburg H (2000a) Correlation of tight junction morphology with the expression of tight junction proteins in blood-brain barrier endothelial cells. Eur J Cell Biol 79:707–717

Liebner S, Fischmann A, Rascher G, Duffner F, Grote E-H, Kalbacher H, Wolberg H (2000b) Claudin-1 and claudin-5 expression and tight junction morphology are altered in blood vessels of human glioblastoma multiforme. Acta Neuropathol 100:323–331

Lindahl P, Johansson BR, Leveen P, Betsholtz C (1997) Pericyte loss and microaneurysm formation in PDGF-B-deficient mice. Science 277:242–245

Lippoldt A, Kniesel U, Liebner S, Kalbacher H, Kirsch T, Wolburg H, Haller H (2000) Structural alterations of tight junctions are associated with loss of polarity in stroke-prone spontaneously hypertensive rat blood-brain barrier endothelial cells. Brain Res 885:251–261

Mamdouh Z, Chen X, Pierini LM, Maxfield FR, Muller WA (2003) Targeted recycling of PECAM from endothelial surface-connected compartments during diapedesis. Nature 421:748–753

Manley GT, Fujimura M, Ma T, Noshita N, Fliz F, Bollen AW, Chan P, Verkman AS (2000). Aquaporin-4 deletion in mice reduces brain edema after acute water intoxication and ischemic stroke. Nature Med 6:159–163

Marcial MA, Carlson SL, Madara JL (1984) Partitioning of paracellular conductance along the ileal crypt-villus axis: a hypothesis based on structural analysis with detailed consideration of tight junction structure-function relationship. J. Membrane Biol 80:59–70

McMahan UJ (1990) The agrin hypothesis. Cold Spring Harbor Symp. Quant. Biol. 55:407–418

Mitic LL, Van Itallie CM, Anderson JM (2000) Molecular physiology and pathophysiology of tight junctions. I. Tight junction structure and function: lessons from mutant animals and proteins. Am J Physiol 279:G250-G254

Morita K, Sasaki H, Furuse M, Tsukita S (1999a) Endothelial claudin: claudin-5/TMVCF constitutes tight junction strands in endothelial cells. J Cell Biol147:185–194

Morita K, Furuse M, Fujimoto K, Tsukita S (1999b) Claudin multigene family encoding four-transmembrane domain protein components of tight junction strands. Proc Natl Acad Sci USA 96:511–516

Nagy Z, Peters H, Hüttner I (1984) Fracture faces of cell junctions in cerebral endothelium during normal and hyperosmotic conditions. Lab. Invest. 50:313–322

Neuhaus J (1990). Orthogonal arrays of particles in astroglial cells: quantitative analysis of their density, size, and correlation with intramembranous particles. Glia 3:241–251.

Nico B, Frigeri A, Nicchia GP, Quondamatteo F, Herken R, Errede M, Ribatti D, Svelto M, Roncali L (2001) Role of aquaporin-4 water channel in the development and integrity of the blood-brain barrier. J Cell Sci 114:1297–1307

Peters A, Palay SL, Webster H (1991) The fine structure of the nervous system, 3rd edn. Oxford University Press, New York

Plumb J, McQuaid S, Mirakhur M, Kirk J (2002) Abnormal endothelial tight junctions in active lesions and normal-appearing white matter in multiple sclerosis. Brain Pathol 12:154–169

Rapoport SI (1976) Blood-brain barrier in physiology and medicine. Raven Press, New York, pp 129–138

Rascher G, Fischmann A, Kröger S, Duffner F, Grote E-H, Wolburg H (2002) Extracellular matrix and the blood-brain barrier in glioblastoma multiforme: spatial segregation of tenascin and agrin. Acta Neuropathol 104:85–91

Reese TS, Karnovsky MJ (1967) Fine structural localization of a blood-brain barrier to exogenous peroxidase. J Cell Biol 34:207–217

Saitou M, Furuse M, Sasaki H, Schulzke J-D, Fromm M, Takano H, Noda T, Tsukita S (2000) Complex phenotype of mice lacking occludin, a component of tight junction strands. Mol Biol Cell 22: 4131–4142.

Sato TN, Tozawa Y, Deutsch U, Wolburg-Buchholz K, Fujiwara Y, Gendron-Maguire M, Gridley T, Wolburg H, Risau W, Qin Y (1995) Distinct roles of the receptor tyrosine kinases tie-1 and tie-2 in blood vessel formation. Nature 376:70–74

Sixt M, Engelhardt B, Pausch F, Hallmann R, Wendler O, Sorokin LM (2001) Endothelial cell laminin isoforms 8 and 10, play decisive roles in T cell recruitment across the blood-brain barrier in experimental autoimmune encephalomyelitis. J Cell Biol 153:933–945

Sobel RA, Hinojoza JR, Maeda A, Chen M (1998) Endothelial cell integrin laminin receptor expression in multiple sclerosis lesions. Am J Pathol 135:405–415

Sims DE (1986) The pericyte – a review. Tissue & Cell 18:153–174

Stanimirovic D, Satoh K (2000) Inflammatory mediators of cerebral endothelium: A role in ischemic brain inflammation. Brain Pathol 10:113–126

Steffen B J, Butcher E C, Engelhardt B (1994) Evidence for involvement of ICAM-1 and VCAM-1 in lymphocyte interaction with endothelium in experimental autoimmune encephalomyelitis in the central nervous system in the SJL/J mouse. Am J Pathol 145:189–201

Tran EH, Hoekstra K, Rooijen NV, Dijkstra CD, Owens T (1998) Immune evasion of the central nervous system parenchyma and experimental allergic encephalomyelitis, but not leukocyte extravasation from blood, are prevented in macrophage-depleted mice. J Immunol 161:3767–3775

Tsukita S, Furuse M, Itoh M (1999) Structural and signalling molecules come together at tight junctions. Curr Op Cell Biol 11:628–633

Vajkoczy P, Laschinger M, Engelhardt B (2001) Alpha4-integrin-VCAM-1 binding mediates G protein-independent capture of encephalitogenic T cell blasts to CNS white matter microvessels. J Clin Invest 108: 557–565

Venero JL, Vizuete ML, Machado A, Cano, J (2001) Aquaporins in the central nervous system. Progr Neurobiol 63:321–336

Vestweber D (2000) Molecular mechanisms that control endothelial cell contacts. J Pathol 190:281–291

von Andrian U H, Engelhardt B (2003) Alpha4 integrins as therapeutic targets in autoimmune disease. N Engl J Med 348:68–72

Weiner HL, Selkoe DJ (2002) Inflammation and therapeutic vaccination in CNS diseases. Nature 420:879–884

Wekerle H, Linington C, Lassmann H, Meyermann R (1986) Cellular immune reactivity within the CNS. Trends Neurosci 9:271–277

Wolburg H (1995) Orthogonal arrays of intramembranous particles. A review with special reference to astrocytes. J Brain Res 36:239–258

Wolburg H, Lippoldt A (2002) Tight junctions of the blood-brain barrier: Development, composition, and regulation. Vascular Pharmacology 38:323–337

Wolburg H, Neuhaus J, Kniesel U, Krauss B, Schmid EM, Öcalan M, Farrell C, Risau W (1994) Modulation of tight junction structure in blood-brain-barrier endothelial-cells–effects of tissue-culture, 2nd messengers and cocultured astrocytes. J Cell Sci 107:1347–1357

Wolburg K, Gerhardt H, Schulz M, Wolburg H, Engelhardt B (1999) Ultrastructural localization of adhesion molecules in the healthy and inflamed choroid plexus of the mouse. Cell Tissue Res 296:259–269

Wolburg H, Wolburg-Buchholz K, Kraus J, Rascher-Eggstein G, Liebner S, Hamm S, Duffner F, Grote E-H, Risau W, Engelhardt B (2003) Localization of claudin-3 in tight junctions of the blood-brain barrier is selectively lost during experimental autoimmune encephalomyelitis and human glioblastoma multiforme. Acta Neuropathol 105:586–592

3 Cytokines in Stroke

S. Allan, C. Stock

3.1 Introduction

Cerebral ischaemia ('stroke') is an acute neurodegenerative disease that is one of the leading causes of death and disability in developed countries. As such it has enormous social as well as financial implications for our society and, despite intense research effort, there is as yet no effective therapy.

There is an increasing awareness that inflammatory processes are important in the brain, particularly in pathophysiological states. Cytokines are a diverse group of polypeptides that have multiple effects on many different cell types. They include the interleukins, interferons, and chemokines as well as the tumour necrosis and growth factors. Cytokines are classically associated with effects in the immune system, but increasing evidence supports a role in both acute and chronic neurodegenerative diseases such as stroke, head injury, and Alzheimer's disease. Since cytokines appear to have a relatively insignificant role in normal physiological function, they may represent an attractive and viable target for new stroke therapies.

The aim of this review therefore is to present evidence supporting a role for cytokines in the pathophysiology of stroke, as well as their possible mechanisms of action. In general the focus will be on those cytokines for which there is the most evidence, i.e. interleukin-1 (IL-1), interleukin-6 (IL-6), tumour necrosis factor-α (TNF-α), and transforming growth factor-β (TGF-β), although other cytokines will be discussed where appropriate.

3.2 Cytokines and Stroke

3.2.1 Overview

The majority of cytokines are present only at very low levels in the normal central nervous system (CNS) but are up-regulated rapidly in response to injury, infection, or inflammation (Quan and Herkenham 2002; Szelenyi 2001).

Cytokines can be classified as either anti-inflammatory or pro-inflammatory. Generally the former are neuroprotective, whereas the latter can contribute to injury and are therefore deemed neurotoxic, although there are exceptions to this (e.g. IL-6). It appears that the exact role of a particular cytokine can depend on a number of different factors, while there is also a large amount of overlap in terms of function between the various cytokines (Quan and Herkenham 2002) (Fig. 1).

A number of lines of evidence have been followed in order to demonstrate a role for cytokines in stroke. These can be broken down into two categories; (1) indirect evidence that is based mainly on experimental studies demonstrating changes in expression in dif-

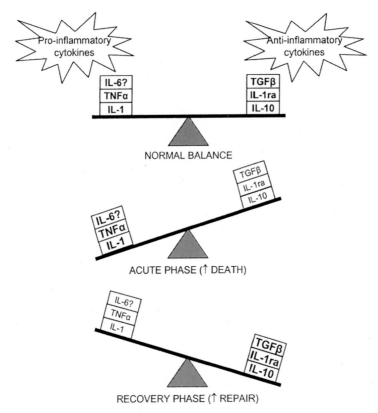

Fig. 1. The contribution of cytokines to outcome in ischaemia depends on a number of different factors, not least of which is the overall balance between anti-inflammatory and pro-inflammatory molecules. A shift in the balance one way or the other will result in either increased or decreased neuronal cell death, depending on which factors dominate, and during which phase

ferent animal models, and where the effects of *exogenous* cytokines on stroke injury have been studied, and (2) direct evidence, gleaned from studies where the effects of inhibiting *endogenous* cytokine action have been investigated. Increasingly, data from studies using transgenic animals contribute to our understanding of the role of cytokines in stroke.

3.2.2 Cytokine Bioactivity and Expression

Regulation of cytokine bioactivity is extremely complex with control exerted at the levels of transcription, translation, and cellular release with additional modulation via soluble binding proteins or receptor antagonists [e.g. IL-1 receptor antagonist (IL-1ra)] and synergistic interactions between cytokines. Furthermore, almost all CNS cell types express most cytokines and their receptors, whilst the mechanisms regulating expression of individual cytokines are closely related (Allan and Rothwell 2001). This multitude of interacting factors not only generates contradictory effects for the same cytokine, it also limits the significance of relationships between expression and functional effect. Thus it may be possible for a cytokine present at very low concentrations overall, but specifically localised and possibly interacting with other cytokines, to exert an effect disproportionate to its gross expression level.

Cytokine expression is induced within the first few h following ischaemic stroke; however there is some confusion over the expression profiles of several cytokines. IL-1β mRNA in rats is increased by 1–2 h after stroke, peaks at 6–12 h before disappearing by 3–5 days (Berti et al. 2002; Buttini et al. 1994; Liu et al. 1993; Zhai et al. 1997). In contrast, IL-1β protein is first detected at 4–6 h and persists until 5–7 days, peaking at 3 days (Davies et al. 1999; Legos et al. 2000). TNF-a and IL-6 mRNAs increase slightly behind IL-1β at 2–3 h post-stroke, peaking at 6 h before declining rapidly over the following 64 h (Ali et al. 2000; Berti et al. 2002; Liu et al. 1994; Zhai et al. 1997). IL-6 protein levels increase at 12 h, peak at 24 h, and are undetectable by 3 days (Legos et al. 2000), whilst TNF-a protein also appears at 12 h but peaks at 3 days, with no detection at 5 days (Sairanen et al. 2001). The discrepancies between mRNA and protein levels of IL-1β, TNF-a and IL-6 are probably indicative of post-transcriptional regulation of cytokine bioactivity. Indeed a number of potential regulatory mechanisms for IL-1 have been described (Watkins et al. 1999). It could also reflect a delay in protein synthesis due to depleted energy stores in ischaemic cells, an observation that is supported by the synchrony between mRNA and protein levels of IL-1ra (Berti et al. 2002; Wang et al. 1997), which is not induced until 12 h post-stroke, when increased cellular energy levels may allow concomitant transcription and translation. Inter-cytokine differences in expression are indicative of their ability to modulate each other's production; for example IL-1 is known to induce its own expression as well as that of IL-6 and TNF-α (Benveniste et al. 1990; Bethea et al. 1992), a fact that is borne out by their respective expression profiles. Similarly, TNF-α promotes IL-6, IL-10 and TGF-β expression, with IL-10 and TGF-β feeding back negatively on TNF-α expression to create an autoregulatory loop as evidenced by identical TNF-α and IL-10 mRNA expression profiles (Benveniste et al. 1990; Chao et al. 1995; Zhai et al. 1997).

The very early induction of cytokines is difficult to explain, especially as it occurs before any histological evidence of cell death. This is thought to preclude microglial cytokine production, which for IL-1 is dependent upon activation of purinergic $P2_X7$ receptors by extracellular ATP released from dying cells (Ferrari et al. 1997). However, it is likely that endothelial and perivascular cells proximal to the infarction point die rapidly, leading to necrosis and possible stimulation of microglia. Furthermore, IL-1β immunoreactive endothelial cells have been observed as early as 15 min after MCA occlusion in the mouse (Zhang et al. 1998), supporting a role for dying endothelia in triggering post-stroke inflammation. Another potential mechanism for cytokine induction is the excitotoxic over-activation of neurones, which has been correlated with increased levels of cytokines during seizures (Jankowsky and Patterson 2001). Similar aberrations in neuronal firing occur early during ischaemia due to neuronal energy depletion, uncontrolled glutamate release, and postsynaptic overactivation (Fisher 1999), and these events may induce IL-1 expression, via an as yet uncharacterised mechanism.

On the whole therefore there is widespread expression of many cytokines in response to an ischaemic insult. Importantly, a number of studies report increased expression before significant cell death is observed, thereby suggesting a causal role in the underlying pathology, rather than simply a response to it.

Cytokine changes in experimental stroke models are supported, in some cases, by clinical findings (Fassbender et al. 1994; Krupinski et al. 1996; Vila et al. 2000). Again the balance between pro- and anti-inflammatory cytokines is probably critical in determining outcome, and this is demonstrated by worse neurological outcome in

ischaemic stroke patients being associated with reduced IL-10 levels
(Vila et al. 2003).

3.2.3 Effects of Recombinant Cytokines

Direct injection of cytokines alone into the brain of normal rodents
does not normally induce brain damage (Quan and Herkenham
2002). This is certainly true for IL-1 (Lawrence et al. 1998),
although direct toxicity is seen with very high concentrations in cortical neuronal cultures, which is in contrast to the protective effects
against excitotoxic cell death seen with lower doses (Strijbos and
Rothwell 1995). In support of this protective role for IL-1, recent
data indicate that excitotoxic cell death is worse in cerebellar granule cell cultures prepared from IL-1RI knockout (KO) mice (Pelidou
et al. 2002). In contrast to these in vitro findings, IL-1 markedly exacerbates brain damage when injected after experimentally induced
ischemia (Loddick et al. 1997; Stroemer and Rothwell 1998; Yamasaki et al. 1995) or excitotoxin administration (Allan et al. 2000;
Lawrence et al. 1998). These conflicting effects of IL-1 are high-
lighted in studies of organotypic slice cultures, when both protective
and toxic actions of IL-1 are seen (Pringle et al. 2001). The reason
for the discrepancies is not clear, although it may depend on a number of factors, including the type of insult and the experimental paradigm, since IL-1 has complex effects on different cell types that
may not be seen in simplified culture systems.

Administration of *exogenous* TNF-α has been shown to induce
cell death in certain in vitro systems, including septo-hippocampal
cultures and PC12 cells (Reimann-Philipp et al. 2001; Zhao et al.
2001). Furthermore, it can induce apoptotic cell death, while inhibiting necrosis, in primary cortical neurones (Reimann-Philipp et al.
2001). These contrasting effects are also observed in vivo, where
TNF-α has been demonstrated to reduce excitotoxic injury (Allan
2002), but exacerbate ischaemic cell death (Barone et al. 1997).

In order to clarify the role of IL-6 in ischaemic injury, Loddick
and colleagues (1998) determined bioactive levels of IL-6 after middle cerebral artery occlusion (MCAo) in the rat. Subsequent experiments then assessed the effect of the same amount of recombinant

IL-6 on MCAo damage, where significant protection was observed (Loddick et al. 1998). Those authors argue therefore that physiologically relevant doses of IL-6 can reduce ischaemic damage and thus *endogenous* IL-6 may be a neuroprotective agent. Support for this comes from both in vitro and in vivo studies demonstrating reduced excitotoxic and ischaemic cell loss in rodents treated with IL-6 (Ali et al. 2000; Matsuda et al. 1996; Toulmond et al. 1992; Yamada and Hatanaka 1993). However, mice with chronic astrocytic overexpression of IL-6 exhibit blood–brain barrier (BBB) breakdown and progressive neurodegenerative disease, which suggests that IL-6 can also have detrimental actions in the CNS (Brett et al. 1995; Campbell et al. 1993). This conflict in IL-6 actions may be related to the cell type expressing IL-6, since neuronal overexpression has no effect on neuronal injury but instead leads to astrogliosis and an increased number of ramified microglia (Fattori et al. 1995).

Similar to application of IL-6, the anti-inflammatory cytokine IL-10 significantly reduces infarct volume following permanent MCAo (Spera et al. 1998), which supports the concept that anti-inflammatory cytokines can be neuroprotective. In this respect, TGF-β reduces both ischaemic and excitotoxic cell death (Henrich-Noack et al. 1995; Prehn et al. 1993).

3.2.4 Inhibition of Cytokine Action

It is important to realise that effects of *exogenous* cytokines do not necessarily represent the function of the *endogenous* molecule, which is often expressed at a low level in a select population of cells. Furthermore, increased production of cytokines may simply reflect the response to neuronal injury rather than active participation in the death process itself. It is important therefore to investigate the contribution of cytokines to stroke thorough modification of the expression, release, or biological activity of the *endogenous* molecule.

Studies of the role of IL-1 in stroke benefit enormously from the availability of IL-1ra, which has no known action other than inhibition of IL-1 (Dinarello and Thompson 1991). The first report on IL-1ra in experimental ischaemia demonstrated that intracerebroventricular administration reduced the infarct resulting from permanent MCAo in the rat by around 60% (Relton and Rothwell 1992). Subsequent studies have confirmed this finding in the rat (Garcia et al. 1995; Loddick and Rothwell 1996; Stroemer and Rothwell 1997) and mouse (Touzani et al. 2002) and have also shown that IL-1ra is effective after both peripheral (Relton et al. 1996) and delayed administration (Ross et al., unpublished data). Other interventions that interfere with *endogenous* IL-1 action, including knockout (Schielke et al. 1998) or inhibition of the IL-1β converting enzyme (Hara et al. 1997; Loddick et al. 1996), administration of neutralising antibody (Yamasaki et al. 1995), and over-expression of IL-1ra (Betz et al. 1995; Yang et al. 1997) also produce a marked reduction in infarct volume resulting from MCAo. In addition, mice deficient in both the IL-1α and IL-1β genes show dramatically reduced ischaemic injury (Boutin et al. 2001), an effect that may be mediated through suppression of oxidative damage (Ohtaki et al. 2003). Support for a role for IL-1 in mediating injury is added to by the finding that IL-1ra is a functional *endogenous* inhibitor of ischaemic cell death, since administration of an anti-IL-1ra antiserum worsens ischaemic injury (Loddick et al. 1997). Given the extensive preclinical data for protective effects of IL-1ra in stroke, and the fact that it has already been demonstrated to be well tolerated in humans (Bresnihan 2001), IL-1ra has entered a Phase II trial for acute cerebral ischaemia (Emsley and Tyrrell 2002). Although IL-1ra does get into the CNS after systemic administration (Gutierrez et al. 1994), whether it proves to be an effective therapy for stroke remains to be seen. Ultimately it may be that smaller-molecule inhibitors of IL-1 represent a better long-term strategy.

Due mainly to the lack of selective inhibitors, there are no studies that have looked directly at the effect on ischaemic damage of blocking *endogenous* IL-6 activity. Furthermore, the use of IL-6 KO mice has provided conflicting data in that neuronal death after cryo-injury is worse in the KO compared to the wild-type mouse (Penkowa et al. 1999), whereas there appears to be no difference with respect to ischaemic injury following MCAo (Clark et al. 2000). However, it may be that the loss of IL-6 is compensated for by other mediators, especially given the extensive overlap in terms of function between different cytokines (Quan and Herkenham 2002).

In contrast to IL-6, there are a number of regulators of *endogenous* TNF-α function available. Administration of soluble TNF receptor, neutralising antibody, or antisense oligonucleotides markedly reduces ischaemic brain damage in the rat (Barone et al. 1997; Mayne et al. 2001; Nawashiro et al. 1996), as does TNF-α-binding protein (Nawashiro et al. 1997). These studies all indicate that endogenous TNF-α directly contributes to neuronal injury. This is in direct conflict to reports suggesting a neuroprotective role in that mice deficient in the p55 or both p55 and p75 TNF receptors show enhanced ischaemic brain damage (Bruce et al. 1996; Gary et al. 1998). However, studies in TNF KO animals indicate that endogenous TNF may indeed have opposing actions on neuronal death in that these animals show improved initial (1–2 days) recovery after traumatic brain injury whilst longer term (2–4 weeks) they have greater neurological dysfunction than the wild-type mice (Scherbel et al. 1999). Thus TNF-α might contribute to early neuronal injury but aid in the repair and recovery process, which would have implications regarding any long-term anti-TNF-α therapy for stroke.

Block of *endogenous* TGF-β with the soluble TGF-β type II receptor exacerbates ischaemic damage in the rat, which supports a neuroprotective role for TGF-β (Ruocco et al. 1999). As yet there have been no studies looking at ischaemic brain injury in TGF-β KO mice, while overexpression of TGF-β leads to severe hydrocephalus and early death, which suggests a possible role for TGF-β in developmental diseases of the CNS (Galbreath et al. 1995) (Table 1).

3.3 Mechanisms of Cytokine Action

3.3.1 Activities related to immune cells

Recruitment of immune cells is the primary function of cytokines in both peripheral and CNS inflammation and is initiated within the first few hours of a stroke occurring. Rapidly induced cytokines such as IL-1 and TNF-α not only activate microglia, but also cause upregulation of adhesion molecules such as intercellular adhesion molecule (ICAM-1/2) by endothelia, which facilitates extravasation of macrophages and neutrophils into the brain parenchyma (Wong and Dorovini-Zis 1992). Despite their vital role in clearing detritus from the ischaemic infarct, the initial effects of immune cell recruit-

Table 1. Major cytokines, their characteristics, and roles in acute cerebral ischaemia

Cytokine	Primary sites of expression and timing (mRNA)	Major targets and receptors	Regulation of bioactivity	Cytokine interactions	Evidence of effects in acute ischaemia	Putative role
IL-1	Microglia, macrophages, and astrocytes 1 h–5 days, peak at 24 h	Endothelia, microglia, astrocytes, macrophages and neurones IL-1RI (effector) IL-1RII (non-func. decoy) ↓ sIL-1RI (soluble decoy) ↓ IL-1ra (Competitive antagonist)	Positive feedback Pro IL-1β must be cleaved by IL-1 converting enzyme (ICE) ↓ sIL-1RI, IL-1RII binding, and IL-1ra antagonism	↑ IL-1, IL-1ra, TNF-α, TGF-β, NGF, and IL-6 expression Synergistic neurotoxicity with TNF-α	↑ Damage with exogenous IL-1β ↓ Damage with IL-1ra ↓ Damage in IL-1$^{-/-}$ mice ↓ Damage when ICE is inhibited Neuroprotective in vitro	Pro-inflammatory and neurotoxic

Table 1 (continued)

Cytokine	Primary sites of expression and timing (mRNA)	Major targets and receptors	Regulation of bioactivity	Cytokine interactions	Evidence of effects in acute ischaemia	Putative role
TNF-α	Microglia, macrophages, and astrocytes; 1 h–5 days, peak at 24 h	Microglia, macrophages, and astrocytes; TNFRI (p55; effector); TNFRII (p75; effector); TBP (soluble antagonist)	Pro TNF-α must be cleaved by TNF-α convertase (TACE/ADAM17) before release; TBP antagonism; Expression inhibited by IL-10 and TGF-β	↑ IL-10, IL-6 and TGF-β expression; Synergistic neurotoxicity with IL-1β	↑ Damage with exogenous TNF-α; ↓ Damage with anti-TNF-α antibody/binding protein; Neuroprotective in vitro	Pro-inflammatory and neurotoxic
TGF-β	Astrocytes and neurones	Microglia, astrocytes, and neurones; TRβ-I/TβR-II (effector complex)	Latent TGF-binding proteins (LTBPs)	↓ TNF-α expression; Possible synergistic neuroprotection with NGF	↓ Damage with exogenous TGF-β; ↑ Damage when endogenous TGF-β is blocked with soluble TbR-II	Anti-inflammatory and neuroprotective

Table 1 (continued)

Cytokine	Primary sites of expression and timing (mRNA)	Major targets and receptors	Regulation of bioactivity	Cytokine interactions	Evidence of effects in acute ischaemia	Putative role
IL-6	Microglia, astrocytes, and macrophages 1–24 h, peak at 6 h	Endothelia, microglia, astrocytes, macrophages, and neurones IL-6R/gp130 (effector complex) sIL-6R (soluble receptor – effector?)	Induction by IL-1 and TNF-α No known endogenous antagonist	Possible induction of neuroprotective NGF	↓ Damage with exogenous IL-6 Neuroprotective against excitotoxicity in vitro IL-6$^{-/-}$ mice can show either no increase or increased damage Constitutively IL-6 over-expressing mice show marked neurodegeneration	Unclear
IL-10	Microglia and astrocytes 4–8 h, peak at 6 h	Microglia, macrophages and astrocytes ↓ IL-10R1 (effector)	↓ Induction by TNF-α	↓ TNF-α expression	↓ Damage with exogenous IL-10 Macrophage de-activation	Anti-inflammatory and neuroprotective

ment promote the progression of injury and cell death. Activated microglia not only upregulate IL-1 secretion in response to ATP 'spilt' from necrotic cells, thus propagating the inflammatory response, but also secrete potentially neurotoxic factors (Giulian et al. 1993; Raivich et al. 1999). The entrapment of circulating leukocytes by adhesion molecules also exacerbates ischaemic damage, mainly by impeding reperfusion of the infarct lesion (del Zoppo et al. 1991). This is illustrated by reduced damage in ICAM KO mice following transient, but not permanent, focal ischaemia and comparable protection following blockade with anti-ICAM antibody (Soriano et al. 1996; Zhang et al. 1994, 1995). Similarly, flushing of the rat brain with saline prior to reperfusion following transient middle cerebral artery occlusion (tMCAo) leads to a significant reduction in damage, correlated with reduced ICAM immunoreactivity (Ding et al. 2002). Although experimental evidence suggested ICAM to be a viable target, when taken into clinical trial anti-ICAM-1 therapy actually worsened outcome (Enlimomab Acute Stroke Trial Investigators 2001).

In addition to an upregulation of endothelial adhesion molecule expression, cytokines have other deleterious effects on vascular function during the acute phase of stroke. IL-1α/β, IL-6, and TNF-α released by perivascular astrocytes increase BBB permeability by opening the tight cell junctions (Abbott 2000, 2002; Mayhan 2001), whilst IL-1β has been implicated in endothelial degradation (Quagliarello et al. 1991). Increases in vascular permeability such as these are key to the development of intracerebral oedema, which contributes to neurological dysfunction and damage progression. In contrast, both IL-1 and IL-6 promote neovascularisation and infiltration of endothelial precursors (Giulian et al. 1988; Swartz et al. 2001), the latter by induction of vascular endothelia growth factor (VEGF) expression in endothelia. These processes are likely to be vital in repairing damaged blood vessels, limiting reperfusion damage and establishing collateral reperfusion during recovery from ischaemia.

3.3.2 Actions on Glia

Neuronal survival and function are heavily dependent on glial cells. However, glia are the primary target of cytokines, and their behaviour is dramatically altered during inflammation. After microglia and infiltrating leukocytes, astrocytes are the main producers and targets of cytokines within the ischaemic brain (Allan and Rothwell 2001). They upregulate expression of a wide range of cytokines in response to IL-1 and TNF-α, including IL-1 and TNF-α themselves, IL-6, and nerve growth factor (NGF). It seems that the overall contribution of cytokines such as IL-1 to neurodegeneration may depend on the extent to which they stimulate differential release of opposing factors such as these. TGF-β also exerts neuroprotective effects through astrocytes by upregulating expression of plasminogen activator inhibitor 1 (PAI 1), which ameliorates NMDA-mediated excitotoxic necrosis (Buisson et al. 1998). However, cytokine-activated astrocytes also form the basis of the glial scar which develops around an ischaemic lesion during recovery (Stoll et al. 1998). Glial scars form a physical barrier to regenerative vascular precursors, axons, oligodendritic processes, and *endogenous* progenitor cells and as such they represent a significant obstacle to regeneration and functional recovery of the infarct zone (Steeves and Tetzlaff 1998; Stoll et al. 1998).

Matrix metalloproteinases (MMPs) are a family of proteolytic enzymes that function to degrade specific target proteins of the extracellular matrix. Increased levels of MMP-9 are seen in stroke patients (Clark et al. 1997) and may contribute to disruption of the BBB as well as acute tissue damage (Gu et al. 2002; Lukes et al. 1999). MMPs are potently regulated by cytokines, particularly in astrocytes, and since they have physiological as well as pathological roles they could act as mediators of both the beneficial and detrimental effects attributed to different cytokines (Gottschall and Yu 1995; Vecil et al. 2000).

3.3.3 Neuronal Effects

The direct actions of cytokines on neurones are poorly characterised in comparison with glial effects. As mention above, IL-1 has been implicated in seizure activity and neurodegeneration caused by intracerebral injection of excitatory substances such as AMPA and kainate (Lawrence et al. 1998; Vezzani et al. 1999, 2000). Other actions of IL-1 on neurones could confer resistance to ischaemia and excitotoxicity such as the inhibition of Ca^{2+} influx and glutamate release seen in vitro, inhibition of long term potentiation (LTP), and enhancement of GABA-mediated synaptic inhibition (O'Connor and Coogan 1999). Similarly TGF-β may protect neurones directly through interaction with NGF, released by astrocytes in response to IL-1 and TNF-α (Yoshida and Gage 1992). On the other hand, it is also likely that IL-1 induces oxidative damage in neurones by upregulation of factors such as inducible nitric oxide synthase (iNOS) and cyclooxygenase (COX-2), which synthesises neurotoxic oxidative species that could contribute to ischaemic damage (Boje and Arora 1992; Nogawa et al. 1997).

IL-1, TNF-α and IL-6 are also potent pyrogens and induce prostaglandin-mediated fever via the hypothalamus (Luheshi and Rothwell 1996), a situation that severely worsens clinical outcome in human stroke patients (Azzimondi et al. 1995; Hajat et al. 2000) and exacerbates ischaemic damage in rodent stroke models (Busto et al. 1987; Morikawa et al. 1992).

3.4 Cytokines and Repair

3.4.1 Background

There is currently great interest in stroke therapies aimed at promoting regeneration and functional recovery. This is largely due to the realisation that CNS neurones are inherently capable of axonal regeneration and that neurogenesis is more common in the adult brain than once thought (Kruger and Morrison 2002). However, the brain is an extremely nonpermissive environment, especially following injury, and recovery-based therapies must address several problems. These problems include combating neurone outgrowth-inhibiting molecules, attenuating formation of a glial scar around the infarct lesion, promoting neurite outgrowth, and improving functional recovery. There are already several promising therapeutic strategies emerging to deal with these problems, such as antibody blockade of inhibitory molecules and cognitive stimulation to facilitate functional recovery (Johansson and Belichenko 2002; Risedal et al. 2002). However, there is also evidence that cytokines may influence these factors, and their effects upon post-stroke recovery need investigation, both to identify any possible therapeutic targets and to assess potential effects of acute-phase anti-inflammatory treatments on the recovery process.

3.4.2 Neurite Outgrowth

Inhibition of neurite outgrowth following CNS injury is largely due to the release of inhibitory molecules, such as Nogo and myelin-associated glycoprotein (MAG), from the inner myelin layers as axons are degraded (Qiu et al. 2000). Microglia and macrophages are responsible for removing necrotic cells and clearing cellular detritus within the infarct zone, including axonal debris and myelin fragments (Qiu et al. 2000; Stoll and Jander 1999). It is possible that acute-phase anti-inflammatory therapies may attenuate this phagocytic response, resulting in higher levels of inhibitory molecules within the lesion due to the persistence of unprocessed axonal debris. This would be of particular importance in cytokine blockade treatments (e.g. IL-1ra) that reduce activation of microglia and leukocytes. On the other hand, IL-1 and TNF-α are responsible for the mobilisation of reactive astrocytes that form glial scars around the lesion site. These scars also inhibit neurite outgrowth via secretion of boundary molecules such as tenascin and chondroitin sulphate proteoglycans (CSPGs), which repulse growing axons (Faissner 1993; McKeon et al. 1991, 1995, 1999). Furthermore, astrocytes and fibrocytes form a physical barrier against regenerative axonal and oligodendritic processes, migrating stem cells, and angiogenic vasculature (Stoll et al. 1998). In addition to boundary molecules, reactive astrocytes release TGF-β into the scar zone, thus propagating scar formation. TGF-β is a key promoter of fibrogenic scarring, and its blockade with anti-TGF-β antibody significantly reduces CNS scar size (Logan et al. 1994), much as it attenuates cutaneous wound scarring (Shah et al. 1994).

Growth factor cytokines such as NGF, foetal growth factor (FGF), insulin-like growth factor (IGF), and brain-derived growth factor (BDGF) promote neurite outgrowth, hippocampal neurogenesis, dendritic sprouting, and synaptic reorganisation (Allan and Rothwell 2001; Nakatomi et al. 2002; Vaillant et al. 2002). These latter two processes are directly associated with neurological plasticity and improved functional recovery in post-ischaemic rats (Johansson and Belichenko 2002). Release of growth factors is in turn dependent on IL-1 and TNF-α activation of glia (Allan and Rothwell 2001), whilst IL-1 and TNF-α expression is also vital for the mobilisation of oligodendrocyte precursor cells. This is demonstrated by reduced oligodendrocyte numbers and impaired remyelination in demyelinated IL-1 and TNF-α KO mice (Arnett et al. 2001; Mason et al. 2001). As mentioned, IL-1 and IL-6 promote neovascularisation (Fee et al. 2000; Zhang et al. 1998), which is essential to reconstructing viable tissue, while IL-6 also promotes proliferation of neuroblastoma cells in vitro (Knezevic-Cuca et al. 2000).

3.4.3 Functional Recovery

In addition to facilitating reconstruction of neural 'hardware' via promotion of neural regeneration and dendritic sprouting, cytokines can have direct effects upon functional recovery. Psychiatric disorders such as depression and reduced motivation are common in stroke patients (Astrom et al. 1992, 1993; Astrom 1996; Berg et al. 2003), and can have severely deleterious effects upon the speed and extent of functional recovery (Gainotti et al. 2001). Cytokines are key components of depressive behaviour (Konsman et al. 2002), and increased levels of circulating cytokines are found in the clinically depressed (Kronfol 2002; Kronfol and Remick 2000). Similarly, rats or mice administered LPS to induce CNS inflammation exhibit sickness behaviour mechanisms, reduced social interaction, and low motivation mediated by IL-1, TNF-α and IL-6. Genetic knockout or blockade of these cytokines attenuates such symptoms (Bluthe et al. 1994, 1995, 2000a,b; Konsman et al. 2002). Together these observations suggest that high cytokine levels (if present during recovery) could impair functional recovery by altering emotional state. Some

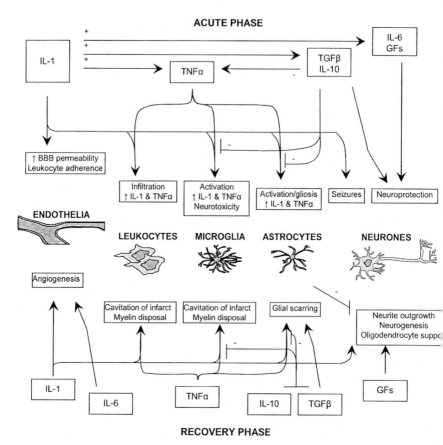

Fig. 2. Schematic diagram to illustrate proposed mechanisms of cytokine action in stroke

cytokines may also have effects upon learning and task acquisition, an important factor in regaining lost functions and motor skills. As mentioned above, cytokines can affect synaptic interactions, and effects of both IL-1 and IL-1ra upon LTP and synaptic reorganisation have been reported (O'Connor and Coogan 1999). It is worth noting that IL-1 KO mice exhibit significant deficits in learning and memory (Goshen et al. 2001), while IL-1ra administration in rats also causes memory impairment (Yirmiya et al. 2002), which is in direct conflict to the finding that IL-1 in rats impairs acquisition of a cognitive task (Aubert et al. 1995) and consolidation of memory (Rachal et al. 2001) (Fig. 2).

3.5 Concluding Remarks

Overall, the effects of cytokines in recovery appear to be just as ambiguous as their roles as mediators of acute damage. Nonetheless, given the difficulties in developing acute therapies for stroke, as indicated by the spectacular list of past failures in clinical trial, it may well be that strategies directed at promoting repair and recovery processes mediated by cytokines in the CNS represent the most logical approach for future stroke treatment.

References

Abbott NJ (2000) Inflammatory mediators and modulation of blood-brain barrier permeability. Cell Mol Neurobiol 20:131–147

Abbott NJ (2002) Astrocyte-endothelial interactions and blood-brain barrier permeability. J Anat 200:629–638

Ali C et al (2000) Ischemia-induced interleukin-6 as a potential endogenous neuroprotective cytokine against NMDA receptor-mediated excitotoxicity in the brain. J Cereb Blood Flow Metab 20:956–966

Allan SM (2002) Varied actions of proinflammatory cytokines on excitotoxic cell death in the rat central nervous system. J Neurosci Res 67:428–434

Allan SM, Parker LC, Collins B, Davies R, Luheshi GN, Rothwell NJ (2000) Cortical cell death induced by interleukin-1 is mediated via actions in the hypothalamus of the rat. Proc Natl Acad Sci USA 97:5580–5585

Allan SM, Rothwell NJ (2001) Cytokines and acute neurodegeneration. Nat Rev Neurosci 2:734–744

Arnett HA, Mason J, Marino M, Suzuki K, Matsushima GK, Ting JP (2001) TNF-alpha promotes proliferation of oligodendrocyte progenitors and remyelination. Nat Neurosci 4:1116–1122

Astrom M (1996) Generalized anxiety disorder in stroke patients. A 3-year longitudinal study. Stroke 27:270–275

Astrom M, Adolfsson R, Asplund K (1993) Major depression in stroke patients. A 3-year longitudinal study. Stroke 24:976–982

Astrom M, Asplund K, Astrom T (1992) Psychosocial function and life satisfaction after stroke. Stroke 23:527–531

Aubert A, Vega C, Dantzer R, Goodall G (1995) Pyrogens specifically disrupt the acquisition of a task involving cognitive processing in the rat. Brain Behav Immun 9:129–148

Azzimondi G et al (1995) Fever in acute stroke worsens prognosis. A prospective study. Stroke 26:2040–2043

Barone FC et al (1997) Tumor necrosis factor-α: A mediator of focal ischemic brain injury. Stroke 28:1233–1244

Benveniste EN, Sparacio SM, Norris JG, Grenett HE, Fuller GM (1990) Induction and regulation of interleukin-6 gene expression in rat astrocytes. J Neuroimmunol 30:201–212

Berg A, Palomaki H, Lehtihalmes M, Lonnqvist J, Kaste M (2003) Poststroke depression: an 18-month follow-up. Stroke 34:138–143

Berti R et al (2002) Quantitative real-time RT-PCR analysis of inflammatory gene expression associated with ischemia-reperfusion brain injury. J Cereb Blood Flow Metab 22:1068–1079

Bethea JR, Chung IY, Sparacio SM, Gillespie GY, Benveniste EN (1992) Interleukin-1-beta induction of tumor necrosis factor-alpha gene expression in human astroglioma cells. J Neuroimmunol 36:179–191

Betz AL, Yang G-Y, Davidson BL (1995) Attenuation of stroke size in rats using an adenoviral vector to induce over expression of interleukin-1 receptor antagonist in brain. J Cerebr Blood Flow Metab 15:547–551

Bluthe RM, Beaudu C, Kelley KW, Dantzer R (1995) Differential effects of IL-1ra on sickness behavior and weight loss induced by IL-1 in rats. Brain Res 677:171–176

Bluthe RM, Laye S, Michaud B, Combe C, Dantzer R, Parnet P (2000a) Role of interleukin-1beta and tumour necrosis factor-alpha in lipopolysaccharide-induced sickness behaviour: a study with interleukin-1 type I receptor-deficient mice. Eur J Neurosci 12:4447–4456

Bluthe RM, Michaud B, Poli V, Dantzer R (2000b) Role of IL-6 in cytokine-induced sickness behavior: a study with IL-6 deficient mice. Physiol Behav 70:367–373

Bluthe RM et al (1994) Synergy between tumor necrosis factor-alpha and interleukin-1 in the induction of sickness behavior in mice. Psychoneuroendocrinol 19:197–207

Boje KM, Arora PK (1992) Microglial-produced nitric oxide and reactive nitrogen oxides mediate neuronal cell death. Brain Res 587:250–256

Boutin H, LeFeuvre RA, Horai R, Asano M, Iwakura Y, Rothwell NJ (2001) Role of IL-1alpha and IL-1beta in ischemic brain damage. J Neurosci 21:5528–5534

Bresnihan B (2001) The safety and efficacy of interleukin-1 receptor antagonist in the treatment of rheumatoid arthritis. Semin Arthritis Rheum 30:17–20

Brett FM, Mizisin AP, Powell HC, Campbell IL (1995) Evolution of neuro-pathologic abnormalities associated with blood-brain barrier breakdown in transgenic mice expressing interleukin-6 in astrocytes. J Neuropathol Exp Neurol 54:766–775

Bruce AJ et al (1996) Altered neuronal and microglial responses to excitotoxic and ischemic brain injury in mice lacking TNF receptors. Nature Med 2:788–794

Buisson A, Nicole O, Docagne F, Sartelet H, MacKenzie ET, Vivien D (1998) Up-regulation of a serine protease inhibitor in astrocytes mediates the neuroprotective activity of transforming growth factor beta1. FASEB J 12:1683–1691

Busto R, Dietrich WD, Globus MY, Valdes I, Scheinberg P, Ginsberg MD (1987) Small differences in intraischemic brain temperature critically determine the extent of ischemic neuronal injury. J Cereb Blood Flow Metab 7:729–738

Buttini M, Sauter A, Boddeke HWGM (1994) Induction of interleukin-1βg mRNA after focal cerebral ischaemia in the rat. Mol Brain Res 23:126–134

Campbell IL et al (1993) Neurologic disease induced in transgenic mice by cerebral overexpression of interleukin 6. Proc Natl Acad Sci USA 90:10061–10065

Chao CC, Hu S, Sheng WS, Tsang M, Peterson PK (1995) Tumor necrosis factor-α mediates the release of bioactive transforming growth factor-β in murine microglial cell cultures. Clin Immunol Immunopathol 77:358–365

Clark AW, Krekoski CA, Bou SS, Chapman KR, Edwards DR (1997) Increased gelatinase A (MMP-2) and gelatinase B (MMP-9) activities in human brain after focal ischemia. Neurosci Lett 238:53–56

Clark WM et al (2000) Lack of interleukin-6 expression is not protective against focal central nervous system ischemia. Stroke 31:1715–1720

Davies CA, Loddick SA, Toulmond S, Stroemer RP, Hunt J, Rothwell NJ (1999) The progression and topographic distribution of interleukin-1beta expression after permanent middle cerebral artery occlusion in the rat. J Cereb Blood Flow Metab 19:87–98

del Zoppo GJ, Schmid-Schonbein GW, Mori E, Copeland BR, Chang CM (1991) Polymorphonuclear leukocytes occlude capillaries following middle cerebral artery occlusion and reperfusion in baboons. Stroke 22:1276–1283

Dinarello CA, Thompson RC (1991) Blocking IL-1: interleukin-1 receptor antagonist in vivo and in vitro. Immunol Today 12:404–410

Ding Y, Li J, Rafols JA, Phillis JW, Diaz FG (2002) Prereperfusion saline infusion into ischemic territory reduces inflammatory injury after transient middle cerebral artery occlusion in rats. Stroke 33:2492–2498

Emsley HC, Tyrrell PJ (2002) Inflammation and infection in clinical stroke. J Cereb Blood Flow Metab 22:1399–1419

Enlimomab Acute Stroke Trial Investigators (2001) Use of anti-ICAM-1 therapy in ischemic stroke: results of the Enlimomab Acute Stroke Trial Neurol 57:1428–1434

Faissner A (1993) Tenascin glycoproteins in neural pattern formation: facets of a complex picture. Perspect Dev Neurobiol 1:155–164

Fassbender K et al (1994) Proinflammatory cytokines in serum of patients with acute cerebral ischemia: kinetics of secretion and relation to the extent of brain damage and outcome of disease. J Neurol Sci 122:135–139

Fattori E, Lazzaro D, Musiani P, Modesti A, Alonzi T, Ciliberto G (1995) IL-6 expression in neurons of transgenic mice causes reactive astrocytosis and increase in ramified microglial cells but no neuronal damage. Eur J Neurosci 7:2441–2449

Fee D et al (2000) Interleukin 6 promotes vasculogenesis of murine brain microvessel endothelial cells. Cytokine 12:655–665

Ferrari D, Chiozzi P, Falzoni S, Hanau S, Di Virgilio F (1997) Purinergic modulation of interleukin-1 beta release from microglial cells stimulated with bacterial endotoxin. J Exp Med 185:579–582

Ferrari D, Los M, Bauer MK, Vandenabeele P, Wesselborg S, Schulze-Osthoff K (1999) P2Z purinoreceptor ligation induces activation of caspases with distinct roles in apoptotic and necrotic alterations of cell death. FEBS Lett 447:71–75

Fisher M (1999) The ischaemic penumbra and the therapeutic window. In: Bogousslavsky, J and Fisher, M. (eds) Current Review of Cerebrovascular Disease, 3rd edn. Current Medicine, Inc., Philadelphia, pp 35–40

Gainotti G, Antonucci G, Marra C, Paolucci S (2001) Relation between depression after stroke, antidepressant therapy, and functional recovery. J Neurol Neurosurg Psychiatry 71:258–261

Galbreath E, Kim SJ, Park K, Brenner M, Messing A (1995) Overexpression of TGF-beta 1 in the central nervous system of transgenic mice results in hydrocephalus. J Neuropathol Exp Neurol 54:339–349

Garcia JH, Liu K-F, Relton JK (1995) Interleukin-1 receptor antagonist decreases the number of necrotic neurons in rats with middle cerebral artery occlusion. Am J Pathol 147:1477–1486

Gary DS, Bruce-Keller AJ, Kindy MS, Mattson MP (1998) Ischemic and excitotoxic brain injury is enhanced in mice lacking the p55 tumor necrosis factor receptor. J Cereb Blood Flow Metab 18:1283–1287

Giulian D, Vaca K, Corpuz M (1993) Brain glia release factors with opposing actions upon neuronal survival. J Neurosci 13:29–37

Giulian D, Woodward J, Young DG, Krebs JF, Lachman LB (1988) Interleukin-1 injected into mammalian brain stimulates astrogliosis and neovascularisation. J Neurosci 8:2485–2490

Goshen I, Avital A, Segal M, Richter-Levin G, Yirmiya R (2001) IL-1 receptor knockout mice display impairments in hippocampal plasticity and memory functions. Brain, Behaviour, and Immunity 15:152

Gottschall PE, Yu X (1995) Cytokines regulate gelatinase A and B (matrix metalloproteinase 2 and 9) activity in cultured rat astrocytes. J Neurochem 64:1513–1520

Gu Z et al (2002) S-nitrosylation of matrix metalloproteinases: signaling pathway to neuronal cell death. Science 297:1186–1190

Gutierrez EG, Banks WA, Kastin AJ (1994) Blood-borne interleukin-1 receptor antagonist crosses the blood-brain barrier. J Neuroimmunol 55:153–160

Hajat C, Hajat S, Sharma P (2000) Effects of poststroke pyrexia on stroke outcome: a meta-analysis of studies in patients. Stroke 31:410–414

Hara H et al (1997) Inhibition of interleukin 1beta converting enzyme family proteases reduces ischemic and excitotoxic neuronal damage. Proc Natl Acad Sci U S A 94:2007–2012

Henrich-Noack P, Krieglstein J, Prehn JHM (1995) TGF-β1 protects hippocampal neurons from ischemic injury: evaluation of potential neuroprotective mechanisms. J Cereb Blood Flow Metab 15:S403

Jankowsky JL, Patterson PH (2001) The role of cytokines and growth factors in seizures and their sequelae. Prog Neurobiol 63:125–149

Johansson BB, Belichenko PV (2002) Neuronal plasticity and dendritic spines: effect of environmental enrichment on intact and postischemic rat brain. J Cereb Blood Flow Metab 22:89–96

Knezevic-Cuca J et al (2000) Neurotrophic role of interleukin-6 and soluble interleukin-6 receptors in N1E-115 neuroblastoma cells. J Neuroimmunol 102:8–16

Konsman JP, Parnet P, Dantzer R (2002) Cytokine-induced sickness behaviour: mechanisms and implications. Trends Neurosci 25:154–159

Kronfol Z (2002) Immune dysregulation in major depression: a critical review of existing evidence. Int.J Neuropsychopharmacol 5:333–343

Kronfol Z, Remick DG (2000) Cytokines and the brain: implications for clinical psychiatry. Am J Psychiatry 157:683–694

Kruger GM, Morrison SJ (2002) Brain repair by endogenous progenitors. Cell 110:399–402

Krupinski J, Kumar P, Kumar S, Kaluza J (1996) Increased expression of TGF-β1 in brain tissue after ischemic stroke in humans. Stroke 27:852–857

Lawrence CB, Allan SM, Rothwell NJ (1998) Interleukin-1beta and the interleukin-1 receptor antagonist act in the striatum to modify excitotoxic brain damage in the rat. Eur J Neurosci 10:1188–1195

Legos JJ, Whitmore RG, Erhardt JA, Parsons AA, Tuma RF, Barone FC (2000) Quantitative changes in interleukin proteins following focal stroke in the rat. Neurosci Lett 282:189–192

Liu T et al (1994) Tumor necrosis factor-a expression in ischemic neurons. Stroke 25:1481–1488

Liu T et al (1993) Interleukin-1β mRNA expression in ischemic rat cortex. Stroke 24:1746–1751

Loddick SA, MacKenzie A, Rothwell NJ (1996) An ICE inhibitor, z-VAD-DCB attenuates ischaemic brain damage in the rat. Neuroreport 7:1465–1468

Loddick SA, Rothwell NJ (1996) Neuroprotective effects of human recombinant interleukin-1 receptor antagonist in focal cerebral ischaemia in the rat. J Cereb Blood Flow Metab 16:932–940

Loddick SA, Turnbull AV, Rothwell NJ (1998) Cerebral interleukin-6 is neuroprotective during permanent focal cerebral ischemia in the rat. J Cereb Blood Flow Metab 18:176–179

Loddick SA, Wong ML, Bongiorno PB, Gold PW, Licinio J, Rothwell NJ (1997) Endogenous interleukin-1 receptor antagonist is neuroprotective. Biochem Biophys ResCommun 234:211–215

Logan A, Berry M, Gonzalez AM, Frautschy SA, Sporn MB, Baird A (1994) Effects of transforming growth factor beta 1 on scar production in the injured central nervous system of the rat. Eur J Neurosci 6:355–363

Luheshi G, Rothwell N (1996) Cytokines and fever. Intl Arch Allerg Immunol 109:301–307

Lukes A, Mun-Bryce S, Lukes M, Rosenberg GA (1999) Extracellular matrix degradation by metalloproteinases and central nervous system diseases. Mol Neurobiol 19:267–284

Mason JL, Suzuki K, Chaplin DD, Matsushima GK (2001) Interleukin-1beta promotes repair of the CNS. J Neurosci 21:7046–7052

Matsuda S et al (1996) Interleukin-6 prevents ischemia-induced learning disability and neuronal and synaptic loss in gerbils. Neurosci Lett 204:109–112

Mayhan WG (2001) Regulation of blood-brain barrier permeability. Microcirc 8:89–104

Mayne M et al (2001) Antisense oligodeoxynucleotide inhibition of tumor necrosis factor-alpha expression is neuroprotective after intracerebral hemorrhage. Stroke 32:240–248

McKeon RJ, Hoke A, Silver J (1995) Injury-induced proteoglycans inhibit the potential for laminin-mediated axon growth on astrocytic scars. Exp Neurol 136:32–43

McKeon RJ, Jurynec MJ, Buck CR (1999) The chondroitin sulfate proteoglycans neurocan and phosphacan are expressed by reactive astrocytes in the chronic CNS glial scar. J Neurosci 19:10778–10788

McKeon RJ, Schreiber RC, Rudge JS, Silver J (1991) Reduction of neurite outgrowth in a model of glial scarring following CNS injury is correlated with the expression of inhibitory molecules on reactive astrocytes. J Neurosci 11:3398–3411

Morikawa E et al (1992) The significance of brain temperature in focal cerebral ischemia: histopathological consequences of middle cerebral artery occlusion in the rat. J Cereb Blood Flow Metab 12:380–389

Nakatomi H et al (2002) Regeneration of hippocampal pyramidal neurons after ischemic brain injury by recruitment of endogenous neural progenitors. Cell 110:429–441

Nawashiro H, Martin D, Hallenbeck JM (1996) Inhibition of tumor necrosis factor and amelioration of brain infarction in mice. J Cereb Blood Flow Metab 17:229–232

Nawashiro H, Martin D, Hallenbeck JM (1997) Neuroprotective effects of TNF binding protein in focal cerebral ischemia. Brain Res 778:265–271

Nogawa S, Zhang F, Ross ME, Iadecola C (1997) Cyclo-oxygenase-2 gene expression in neurons contributes to ischemic brain damage. J Neurosci 17:2746–2755

O'Connor JJ, Coogan AN (1999) Actions of the pro-inflammatory cytokine IL-1β on central synaptic transmission. Exp Physiol 84:601–614

Ohtaki H et al (2003) Suppression of oxidative neuronal damage after transient middle cerebral artery occlusion in mice lacking interlekin-1. Neurosci Res 45:313–324

Pelidou SH, Schultzberg M, Iverfeldt K (2002) Increased sensitivity to N-methyl-D-aspartate receptor-induced excitotoxicity in cerebellar granule cells from interleukin-1 receptor type I-deficient mice. J Neuroimmunol 133:108–115

Penkowa M et al (1999) Strongly compromised inflammatory response to brain injury in interleukin-6-deficient mice. Glia 25:343–357

Prehn JH, Backhauss C, Krieglstein J (1993) Transforming growth factor-beta 1 prevents glutamate neurotoxicity in rat neocortical cultures and protects mouse neocortex from ischemic injury in vivo. J Cereb Blood Flow Metab 13:521–525

Pringle AK, Niyadurupola N, Johns P, Anthony DC, Iannotti F (2001) Interleukin-1beta exacerbates hypoxia-induced neuronal damage, but attenuates toxicity produced by simulated ischaemia and excitotoxicity in rat organotypic hippocampal slice cultures. Neurosci Lett 305:29–32

Qiu J, Cai D, Filbin MT (2000) Glial inhibition of nerve regeneration in the mature mammalian CNS. Glia 29:166–174

Quagliarello VJ, Wispelwey B, Long Jr WJ, Scheld WM (1991) Recombinant human interleukin-1 induces meningitis and blood-brain barrier injury in the rat. Characterization and comparison with tumor necrosis factor. J Clin Invest 87:1360–1366

Quan N, Herkenham M (2002) Connecting cytokines and brain: a review of current issues. Histol Histopathol 17:273–288

Rachal PC, Fleshner M, Watkins LR, Maier SF, Rudy JW (2001) The immune system and memory consolidation: a role for the cytokine IL-1beta. Neurosci Biobehav Rev 25:29–41

Raivich G, Bohatschek M, Kloss CU, Werner A, Jones LL, Kreutzberg GW (1999) Neuroglial activation repertoire in the injured brain: graded response, molecular mechanisms and cues to physiological function. Brain Res Brain Res Rev 30:77–105

Reimann-Philipp U, Ovase R, Weigel PH, Grammas P (2001) Mechanisms of cell death in primary cortical neurons and PC12 cells. J Neurosci Res 64:654–660

Relton JK, Martin D, Thompson RC, Russell DA (1996) Peripheral administration of interleukin-1 receptor antagonist inhibits brain damage after focal cerebral ischemia in the rat. Exp Neurol 138:206–213

Relton JK, Rothwell NJ (1992) Interleukin-1 receptor antagonist inhibits ischaemic and excitotoxic neuronal damage in the rat. Brain Res Bull 29:243–246

Risedal A, Mattsson B, Dahlqvist P, Nordborg C, Olsson T, Johansson BB (2002) Environmental influences on functional outcome after a cortical infarct in the rat. Brain Res Bull 58:315–321

Ruocco A et al (1999) A transforming growth factor-beta antagonist unmasks the neuroprotective role of this endogenous cytokine in excitotoxic and ischemic brain injury. J Cereb Blood Flow Metab 19:1345–1353

Sairanen T et al (2001) Evolution of cerebral tumor necrosis factor-alpha production during human ischemic stroke. Stroke 32:1750–1758

Scherbel U et al (1999) Differential acute and chronic responses of tumor necrosis factor-α deficient mice to experimental brain injury. Proc Natl Acad Sci USA 96:8721–8726

Schielke GP, Yang GY, Shivers BD, Betz AL (1998) Reduced ischemic brain injury in interleukin-1 beta converting enzyme-deficient mice. J Cereb Blood Flow Metab 18:180–185

Shah M, Foreman DM, Ferguson MW (1994) Neutralising antibody to TGF-beta 1,2 reduces cutaneous scarring in adult rodents. J Cell Sci 107 (Pt 5):1137–1157

Soriano SG et al (1996) Intercellular adhesion molecule-1-deficient mice are less susceptible to cerebral ischemia-reperfusion injury. Ann Neurol 39:618–624

Spera PA, Ellison JA, Feuerstein GZ, Barone FC (1998) IL-10 reduces rat brain injury following focal stroke. Neurosci Lett 251:189–192

Steeves JD, Tetzlaff W (1998) Engines, accelerators, and brakes on functional spinal cord repair. Ann NY Acad Sci 860:412–424

Stoll G, Jander S (1999) The role of microglia and macrophages in the pathophysiology of the CNS. Prog Neurobiol 58:233–247

Stoll G, Jander S, Schroeter M (1998) Inflammation and glial responses in ischemic brain lesions. Prog Neurobiol 56:149–171

Strijbos PJLM, Rothwell NJ (1995) Interleukin-1β attenuates excitatory amino acid-induced neurodegeneration in vitro: involvement of nerve growth factor. JNeurosci 15:3468–3474

Stroemer RP, Rothwell NJ (1997) Cortical protection by localized striatal injection of IL-1ra following cerebral ischemia in the rat. J Cereb Blood Flow Metab 17:597–604

Stroemer RP, Rothwell NJ (1998) Exacerbation of ischemic brain damage by localized striatal injection of interleukin-1beta in the rat. J Cereb Blood Flow Metab 18:833–839

Swartz KR et al (2001) Interleukin-6 promotes post-traumatic healing in the central nervous system. Brain Res 896:86–95

Szelenyi J (2001) Cytokines and the central nervous system. Brain Res Bull 54:329–338

Toulmond S, Fage VD, Benavides J (1992) Local infusion of interleukin-6 attenuates the neurotoxic effects of NMDA on rat striatal cholinergic neurons. Neurosci Lett 144:49–52

Touzani O et al (2002) Interleukin-1 influences ischemic brain damage in the mouse independently of the interleukin-1 type I receptor. J Neurosci 22:38–43

Vaillant AR, Zanassi P, Walsh GS, Aumont A, Alonso A, Miller FD (2002) Signaling mechanisms underlying reversible, activity-dependent dendrite formation. Neuron 34:985–998

Vecil GG et al (2000) Interleukin-1 is a key regulator of matrix metalloproteinase-9 expression in human neurons in culture and following mouse brain trauma in vivo. J Neurosci Res 61:212–224

Vezzani A et al (1999) Interleukin-1β immunoreactivity and microglia are enhanced in the rat hippocampus by focal kainate application: functional evidence for enhancement of electrographic seizures. J Neurosci 19:5054–5065

Vezzani A et al (2000) Powerful anticonvulsant action of IL-1 receptor antagonist on intracerebral injection and astrocytic overexpression in mice. Proc Natl Acad Sci USA 97:11534–11539

Vila N, Castillo J, Davalos A, Chamorro A (2000) Proinflammatory cytokines and early neurological worsening in ischemic stroke. Stroke 31:2325–2329

Vila N, Castillo J, Davalos A, Esteve A, Planas AM, Chamorro A (2003) Levels of anti-inflammatory cytokines and neurological worsening in acute ischemic stroke. Stroke 34:671–675

Wang X, Barone FC, Aiyar NV, Feuerstein GZ (1997) Interleukin-1 receptor and receptor antagonist gene expression after focal stroke in rats. Stroke 28:155–162

Watkins LR, Hansen MK, Nguyen KT, Lee JE, Maier SF (1999) Dynamic regulation of the proinflammatory cytokine, interleukin-1β: molecular biology for non-molecular biologists. Life Sci 65:449–481

Wong D, Dorovini-Zis K (1992) Upregulation of intercellular adhesion molecule-1 (ICAM-1) expression in primary cultures of human brain microvessel endothelial cells by cytokines and lipopolysaccharide. J Neuroimmunol 39:11–21

Yamada M, Hatanaka H (1993) Interleukin-6 protects cultured rat hippocampal neurons against glutamate-induced cell death. Brain Res 643:173–180

Yamasaki Y, Matsuura N, Shozuhara H, Onodera H, Itoyama Y, Kogure K (1995) Interleukin-1 as a pathogenetic mediator of ischemic brain damage in rats. Stroke 26:676–681

Yang G-Y, Zhao Y-J, Davidson BL, Betz AL (1997) Overexpression of interleukin-1 receptor antagonist in the mouse brain reduces ischemic brain injury. Brain Res 751:181–188

Yirmiya R, Winocur G, Goshen I (2002) Brain interleukin-1 is involved in spatial memory and passive avoidance conditioning. Neurobiol Learn Mem 78:379–389

Yoshida K, Gage FH (1992) Cooperative regulation of nerve growth factor synthesis and secretion in fibroblasts and astrocytes by fibroblast growth factor and other cytokines. Brain Res 569:14–25

Zhai Q-H, Futrell N, Chen F-J (1997) Gene expression of IL-10 in relationship to TNF-α, IL-1β and IL-2 in the rat brain following middle cerebral artery occlusion. J Neurol Sci 152:119–124

Zhang RL et al (1995) Anti-intercellular adhesion molecule-1 antibody reduces ischemic cell damage after transient but not permanent middle cerebral artery occlusion in the Wistar rat. Stroke 26:1438–1443

Zhang RL et al (1994) Anti-ICAM-1 antibody reduces ischemic cell damage after transient middle cerebral artery occlusion in the rat. Neurol 44:1747–1751

Zhang Z, Chopp M, Goussev A, Powers C (1998) Cerebral vessels express interleukin 1β after focal cerebral ischemia. Brain Res 784:210–217

Zhao X et al (2001) TNF-alpha stimulates caspase-3 activation and apoptotic cell death in primary septo-hippocampal cultures. J Neurosci Res 64: 121–131

4 Complement Activation: Beneficial and Detrimental Effects in the CNS

J. van Beek

4.1 The Complement System, an Important Effector of the Innate Immune Response

Functions of the complement system include the recognition and killing of invading pathogens (e.g., bacteria, virus-infected cells, parasites) while preserving normal "self" cells. The complement system also contributes through its activation to the release of inflammatory mediators, promoting potential tissue injury at sites of inflammation (Frank and Fries 1991). Having preceded the emergence of adaptive immunity, the complement system has maintained a high

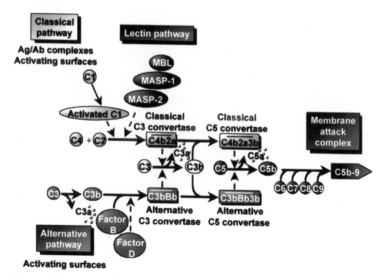

Fig. 1. Schematic representation of the complement cascade. The complement system can be activated through the classical, the alternative, or the lectin pathway, leading to a common terminal pathway: the cytolytic membrane attack complex (MAC). Proteolytic cleavage of components C3 and C5 leads to the release of pro-inflammatory anaphylatoxins C3a and C5a, respectively. *MBL*, mannose-binding lectin; *MASP*, MBL-associated serine protease; *Ag*, antigen; *Ab*, antibody

degree of phylogenic conservation among both invertebrates and mammals, underlying the critical role of complement in tissue homeostasis (Sunyer et al. 1998).

The complement system consists of some 30 fluid-phase and cell-membrane-associated proteins. Complement can be activated by three distinct routes (Fig. 1). The classical pathway (involving C1q, C1r, C1s, C4, C2, and C3 components) is activated primarily by the interaction of C1q with immune complexes (antibody-antigen), but activation can also be achieved after interaction of C1q with nonimmune molecules such as DNA, RNA, C-reactive protein, serum amyloid P, bacterial lipopolysaccharides, and some fungal and virus membranes. The initiation of the alternative pathway (involving C3, factor B, factor D, and properdin) does not require the presence of immune complexes and leads to the deposition of C3 fragments on target cells. Mannose-binding lectin (MBL), a lectin homologous to C1q, can recognize carbohydrates such as mannose and *N*-acetylglucosamine on pathogens and initiate the complement pathway independently of both the classical and alternative activation pathways. MBL is associated with two serine-proteases, mannose-binding lectin-associated serine proteases (MASP)-1 and 2, that, like the C1 complex in the classical pathway, cleave C4 and C2 components, leading to the formation of the classical C3 convertase.

4.2 Complement Receptors Involved in Phagocytosis

The target pathogen coated with complement opsonins (C1q and C3 activation by-products: C3b, iC3b) is specifically recognized and phagocytosed by macrophages expressing complement C1q and receptors for C3 fragments [complement receptor (CR) type 1, CR3, and CR4]. In addition to its role in pathogen clearance, C1q has been shown to play an important role in the clearance of apoptotic cells. C1q binds directly to surface blebs of apoptotic keratinocytes and T cells, and there can initiate complement opsonisation (Botto et al. 1998; Taylor et al. 2000). These observations strongly support the hypothesis that C1q serves as an opsonin in the recognition and clearance of apoptotic cells. The transmembrane glycoprotein termed "C1q receptor that enhances phagocytosis" (C1qRp), recently shown to be identical to CD93, has emerged as a possible defense collagen receptor (McGreal et al. 2002). Monocytes that have adhered on C1q-coated surfaces display a four- to tenfold enhancement of phagocytosis of targets coated with IgG or complement (Guan et al. 1994). However, the alleged binding of C1q to CD93 has been challenged, and the cellular and molecular properties of the multicomplex receptor CD93 are yet to be elucidated (McGreal et al. 2002).

C3, when activated on a cell surface, binds covalently (opsonisation) as C3b and is subsequently cleaved into a very stable fragment iC3b. CR3 (CD11b/CD18) and CR4 (CD11c/CD18) are involved in the phagocytosis process of targets opsonized with C3b and iC3b fragments (Ehlers 2000). CR1 (CD35) is also a multifunctional receptor binding to C4b, C3b, iC3b, and C1q, and as such has been implicated in phagocytic and complement regulatory activities (Krych-Goldberg and Atkinson 2001).

4.3 The Lytic Terminal Complex and Complement Regulators

Ultimately, activation of the complement system leads to the formation, through the complement terminal pathway (involving C5, C6, C7, C8, and C9 components), of the membrane attack complex (MAC) which forms a pore in the phospholipid bilayer to lyse the target cell (i.e., bacteria or virally infected cells). However, activa-

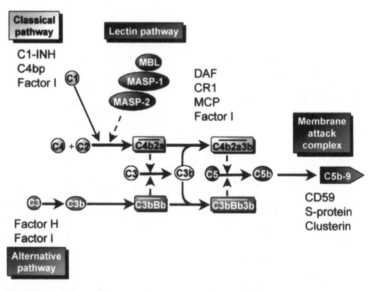

Fig. 2. Regulation of the complement cascade. The different pathways of the complement cascade are tightly regulated by membrane-associated (DAF, MCP, CD59, CR1) or soluble (C1-INH, C4 bp, Factor I, Factor H, S-protein, clusterin) inhibitors. *C1-INH*, C1 inhibitor; *C4 bp*, C4 binding protein; *DAF*, decay-accelerating factor; *MCP*, membrane cofactor protein; *CR1*, complement receptor 1

tion of the complement system at inappropriate sites and/or to an inappropriate extent can lead to host tissue damage.

To protect 'self' cells against by-stander lysis, host cells express a battery of regulatory proteins (complement inhibitors) which inhibit either assembly of the C3-cleaving enzymes or the formation of the MAC (Fig. 2; Morgan and Harris 1999). C1 inhibitor (C1-INH), C4 binding protein (C4 bp), factor H, factor I, S-protein, and clusterin are soluble inhibitors secreted and released in the fluid phase. Membrane-associated complement inhibitors include membrane cofactor protein (MCP, CD46), decay-accelerating factor (DAF, CD55), and CD59. Of note, an inhibitor of complement activation termed "complement receptor-related protein y" (Crry) is expressed on rodent, but not human, cell membranes. Crry is broadly distributed and is a functional and structural analogue of human DAF and MCP.

4.4 Complement Expression by Brain Cells

In mammals, the liver is the major source of most complement proteins with the exception of C1q, C7, and FD. The brain is separated from the plasma by the blood–brain barrier (BBB), formed by endothelial cells of microvessels, smooth muscle cells (also called pericytes), and astrocytes. The BBB acts as a molecular sieve and isolates the brain parenchyma from plasma proteins, including complement components, as well as circulating immunocompetent cells such as lymphocytes, macrophages, and natural killer cells. However, transudation of plasma proteins through a damaged BBB can contribute to the deposition of potentially cytotoxic and cytolytic complement components in the brain parenchyma.

In addition, we and others have proposed that brain cells can produce complement proteins to recognize and kill pathogens locally while preserving normal cells in the central nervous system (CNS) (Morgan and Gasque 1996). Levi-Strauss and Mallat (1987) were the first to demonstrate that brain cells can synthesize complement components. They showed that cultured rodent astrocyte cell lines and primary cultures of mouse astrocytes produced C3 and FB, and that the expression of complement was increased upon stimulation with lipopolysaccharide (LPS). In the last decade, this observation has been extended to include astrocytes, microglia, neurones, and oligodendrocytes (Barnum 1995; Gasque et al. 2000). Cell lines and primary cultures of human origin were used to show that glial and neuronal cells were able to produce most complement proteins, particularly after stimulation with inflammatory cytokines (Gasque et al. 1992, 1993, 1995; Thomas et al. 2000). Complement mRNAs were also found to be expressed, albeit at a low level, in normal human brain tissue (Witte et al. 1991; Walker and McGeer 1992; Fischer et al. 1995; Shen et al. 1997; Yasojima et al. 1999a, b). From these studies, it was proposed that brain cells, appropriately stimulated with cytokines, can assemble a full complement system to exert toxic and lytic activities against pathogens.

In addition, there is now considerable evidence that local expression of complement by resident cells can be dramatically increased following brain infection. Increased levels of complement mRNAs have been reported in experimental models of brain infection (meningitis, scrapie, encephalomyelitis) in rodents (Dietzschold et al. 1995; Stahel et al. 1997a, b; Dandoy-Dron et al. 1998).

4.5 Complement in Acute Brain Inflammation: Cerebral Ischemia and Trauma

After an acute brain insult, such as a stroke or traumatic brain injury, local inflammation within the brain parenchyma can contribute to the exacerbation of neuronal loss. The concept that complement activation may contribute to the pathogenesis of acute brain injury developed from observations using experimental models of stroke and trauma. Systemic complement depletion using cobra venom factor (CVF), which functions as an unregulated C3 convertase, thus activating and depleting C3 and C5 via the alternative pathway, was found to improve blood flow and neurological function after transient cerebral ischemia in the rat (Vasthare et al. 1998). Huang and colleagues (1999) demonstrated that a bifunctional molecule designed to inhibit both complement activation and selectin-mediated adhesive events can inhibit neutrophil and platelet accumulation and reduce cerebral infarct size in the mouse. Furthermore, treatment with soluble CR1 was found to reduce neutrophil accumulation after traumatic brain injury in rats (Kaczorowski et al. 1995). More recently, the effect of C1-INH, the only known inhibitor of complement C1, was investigated in a murine model of transient focal ischemia (De Simoni et al. 2003). In this model, C1-INH significantly improved general and focal deficits, and significantly reduced infarct volume.

The presence of complement components within the brain parenchyma following experimental cerebral ischemia has been documented. Intracerebral complement levels following acute brain injury might increase after BBB breakdown, leading to passive leakage of serum-derived complement into the brain parenchyma. In 1994, Czurko and Nishino reported the presence of C3, along with the infiltration of immunoglobulins, within both the striatum and the cortex following transient focal cerebral ischemia in the rat (Czurko and Nishimo 1994). Additionally, potential cellular sources of complement within the injured brain have been identified. Using in situ hybridization, widespread increased synthesis of C1q was found in microglial cells in response to transient global cerebral ischemia in rats (Schafer et al. 2000). Intracerebral expression of complement following focal cerebral ischemia was mainly associated with the glial cell response but neurons can also be a source of complement (van Beek et al. 2000a). Local complement production has also been described in experimental models of trauma. For instance, expression of mRNA for C1q was found in the peritrauma region after a cortical aspiration lesion in rats (Pasinetti et al. 1992). Deposition of the complement activation product C3d and C9, an indicator of MAC deposition, was observed on neurones following experimental cerebral contusion in the rat (Bellander et al. 1996).

In line with these findings in experimental models are reports of intrathecal synthesis of complement, as assessed by the presence of several activation products of the cytotoxic/cytolytic complement system in the cerebrospinal fluid (CSF) of head trauma or stroke patients. In these studies, elevated levels of complement components C3 and factor B were found in ventricular CSF of patients with traumatic brain injury (Stahel et al. 1997c). Interestingly, intrathecal levels of complement-derived soluble MAC correlate with BBB dysfunction, implicating the complement system in the pathogenesis of clinical trauma, with regard to post-traumatic BBB dysfunction

(Stahel et al. 2001). Complement activation in CSF and plasma following cerebral ischemia or hemorrhage has also been reported (Kasuya and Shimizu, 1989; Lindsberg et al. 1996).

Strikingly, complement activation products have been localized within the CNS parenchyma of head trauma (Bellander et al. 2001) and of patients with subarachnoid hemorrhage or brain infarction (Lindsberg et al. 1996), providing a strong body of evidence that complement-mediated cell death is prominent in areas of brain damage. Xiong and colleagues recently reported direct evidence for deleterious consequences of MAC deposition in the brain. Sequential infusion of individual proteins of the MAC (C5b6, C7, C8, and C9) into the hippocampus of awake rats induced both behavioral and electrographic seizures, as well as cytotoxicity (Xiong et al. 2003).

4.6 Neurones are Susceptible to Complement Attack

Brain cells such as astrocytes and microglia express complement inhibitors to control complement activation on their membranes, and seem to be relatively well protected from complement-mediated damage. This is in sharp contrast to neurones, which are extremely susceptible to complement attack. Indeed, human neuroblastoma cells as well as embryonic neurones in vitro have the propensity to activate spontaneously the complement system and, consequently, are susceptible to complement-mediated lysis (Gasque et al. 1996; Singhrao et al. 2000). C1q binds specifically to the membrane of neurones, leading to the activation of the classical pathway in an antibody-independent manner. The poor capacity of neurones to control complement activation has been attributed to the fact that these cells express low levels of complement regulators (Singhrao et al. 1999 a, b). Overall, there is now considerable evidence that increased intracerebral complement biosynthesis and uncontrolled complement activation in the CNS contribute to the development of tissue damage. However, further data on complement activation in stroke and trauma patients are needed before suggesting the possibility of a pharmacological manipulation of the complement system in acute brain injury (del Zoppo 1999; Di Napoli 2001).

4.7 Complement Anaphylatoxins and Their Receptors

The most potent inflammatory molecules generated upon complement activation are the anaphylatoxins C3a and C5a. C3a and C5a are small polypeptides (~9–10 kDa) that are highly pleiotropic in function and exert their effect at picomolar to nanomolar concentrations (Ember et al. 1998). C3a and C5a derive from the enzymatic cleavage of C3 and C5 respectively and are involved in the stimulation and chemotaxis of myeloid cells. The functional responses induced by C3a and C5a are mediated through their binding to specific receptors, C3a and C5a receptors (C3aR and C5aR), respectively (Ember et al. 1998). These receptors are members of the rhodopsin family of seven transmembrane G-protein-coupled receptors (Boulay et al. 1991; Gerard and Gerard, 1991; Ames et al. 1996; Crass et al. 1996; Roglic et al. 1996).

C5a is an important chemoattractant molecule and stimulates cells to express increased levels of cytokines, chemokines, adhesion molecules, and complement components (Ember et al. 1998). In contrast to the broad pro-inflammatory effects of C5a, the effects of C3a appear to be more selective and rather anti-inflammatory. C3a is chemoattractant but only for mast cells and eosinophils and not for macrophages or microglia. Recent data indicate that C3a can decrease the production of pro-inflammatory cytokines by LPS-stimulated macrophages and, on the other hand, can induce the production of immunosuppressive cytokines such as IL-10 (Ember et al. 1998). Furthermore, mice with targeted disruption of C3aR exhibited an enhanced lethality when subjected to endotoxin shock, underlying the potential anti-inflammatory properties of anaphylatoxin C3a (Kildsgaard et al. 2000).

The expression of C3aR and C5aR was thought to be restricted largely to cells of the myeloid lineage such as macrophages, eosinophils, basophils, and mast cells (Daffern et al. 1995; Martin et al. 1997; Zwirner et al. 1999). However, in recent years, studies have reported widespread expression of these receptors throughout many tissues and cell types outside the immune system, supporting the view that anaphylatoxins might even exert effects unrelated to inflammation (Wetsel 1995; Ember and Hugli 1997; Zwirner et al. 1999). If the presence of C3aR and C5aR on microglia was expected given the monocytic origin of these cells, their expression on astrocytes and neurones was not anticipated. The functional significance of the presence of anaphylatoxin receptors on neurones remains ill-defined, but preliminary work suggests that anaphylatoxins might be involved in the modulation of neuronal functions (Nataf et al. 1999).

Upregulated expression of anaphylatoxin receptors by brain cells has been described in experimental models of focal cerebral ischemia (van Beek et al. 2000b; Barnum et al. 2002) and trauma (Stahel et al. 1997b, 2000), suggesting a role for anaphylatoxins in the pathogenesis of acute brain injury. Human astrocyte cell lines stimulated with C5a produce increased amounts of IL-6, whereas the levels of IL-1, TNF-α and TGF-β remain unchanged (Sayah et al. 1999). Unexpectedly, C5a has been shown to induce apoptosis of the human neuroblastoma cell line TGW (Farkas et al. 1998a,b). Taken together, these data suggest that C5a release during CNS inflammation could contribute to the exacerbation of tissue damage. However, protective roles of C5a cannot be excluded, because anaphylatoxin C5a has been shown to protect neurones against excitotoxicity (Osaka 1999a,b; Mukherjee and Pasinetti 2001). Interestingly, Heese and colleagues (1998) have shown that a human microglial cell line exposed to C3a expressed de novo nerve growth factor (NGF), a molecule involved in neuronal growth and survival. These data would support the view that C3a, in contrast to C5a, acts as an anti-inflammatory signal promoting the resolution of the inflammatory process. Unlike C5a, C3a failed to display any effect on apoptosis-mediated neuronal cell death; however, C3a was shown to protect neurones against N-methyl-D-aspartate toxicity, extending its role beyond immune functions (van Beek et al. 2001). Further studies to investigate the role of complement anaphylatoxins in the modulation of neuroprotective/neurotoxic pathways are warranted.

4.8 Sublytic Effects of MAC

Assembly of the MAC is, by definition, involved in cytolytic activities. However, when the number of MAC molecules is limited, cells are able to escape cell death by rapidly eliminating membrane-inserted MAC by endocytosis and membrane shedding (Morgan 1989). When it does not cause death, the MAC is involved in cell stimulation (Morgan 1989; Rus et al. 2001). Sublytic levels of MAC have been shown to increase Ca^{2+} influx, to activate phospholipases and protein kinases, and to induce the generation of arachidonic acid-derived inflammatory mediator (Imagawa et al. 1983; Wiedmer et al. 1987; Niculescu et al. 1993; Shirazi et al. 1987; Carney et al. 1990). The MAC at the sublytic level has also been shown to stimulate endothelial cells to express complement regulatory proteins and to protect against secondary damage (Mason et al. 1999). Taken together, these data indicate that the MAC at the sublytic level could act as a stress signal to activate cells to express increased levels of complement inhibitors and protect against subsequent damage.

As an example of the protective role of MAC, postmitotic oligodendrocytes exposed to sublytic MAC have been shown to enter the cell cycle (Rus et al. 1996, 1997). Moreover, exposure to sublytic MAC has been demonstrated to protect oligodendrocytes from apoptosis induced by serum deprivation (Rus et al. 1996) or exposure to tumor necrosis factor-a (Soane et al. 1999). The question of whether sublytic assembly of the MAC could also modulate the outcome of damage during the course of demyelinating disease was addressed recently using experimental allergic encephalomyelitis. C5-sufficient mice with EAE were found to develop less pronounced levels of inflammation compared to C5-deficient mice, unable to form the MAC (Rus et al. 2002). In addition, active remyelination with restoration of tissue integrity was observed in chronic lesions only in C5-sufficient mice (Rus et al. 2002). Taken together, these data suggest a possible role for the sublytic assembly of MAC in the modulation of tissue inflammation and the initiation of tissue repair.

4.9 Conclusion

Given the multiple functions of the complement system, it has been difficult thus far to identify their specific roles in the pathogenesis of CNS disorders. Although there is a wealth of data implicating the complement system in the propagation of brain inflammation and tissue injury, the possibility that complement is involved in neuro-

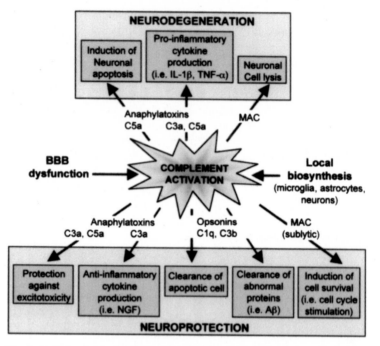

Fig. 3. Complement activation within the CNS: a double edged-sword. Complement components found in the brain parenchyma under pathological conditions can originate either from the plasma after blood–brain barrier (BBB) dysfunction or from local biosynthesis by activated brain cells. Intracerebral complement activation may promote tissue damage by inducing neuronal cell death (anaphylatoxins and MAC) and by promoting the release of pro-inflammatory cytokines by activated glial cells. On the other hand, complement activation can exert beneficial effects on the brain by promoting neuroprotection (anaphylatoxins, sublytic MAC) and tissue remodeling (opsonins and anaphylatoxins)

protective and repair activities is emerging. These double-edged sword activities of the local innate complement system in the CNS are summarized in Fig. 3.

The case for an important role of complement in the initiation and/or exacerbation of brain inflammation has implications for therapeutic strategies to prevent secondary tissue injury. Complement therapeutics have undergone a mini-revolution over the last decade with the development of agents, based upon the naturally occurring regulators of complement, that efficiently inhibit complement when administered to animals or humans (Morgan 1996). As noted earlier, some of these agents (e.g., complement inhibitor C1-INH) have been shown to markedly reduce brain inflammation and tissue damage (De Simoni et al. 2003). However, none of the current crop of complement therapeutics is suited to treatment of a chronic disease. All are large molecules, active only when administered systemically, and they have relatively short half-lives. These shortcomings effectively restrict use to acute disorders. Furthermore, in order to be used in CNS diseases, the next generation of complement inhibitors will have to be designed so that they can be specifically delivered to the brain (by the use of specific targeting moieties) or expressed in the brain (by gene therapy).

Since many of the responses mediated by the complement system can lead to beneficial effects, directing activation of the complement system, rather than inhibiting it, might inaugurate the basis for the development of new complement therapeutics.

Acknowledgements. Philippe Gasque and B. Paul Morgan are acknowledged for their helpful comments on the manuscript. This work was supported by the Wellcome Trust.

References

Ames RS, Li Y, Sarau HM, Nuthulaganti P, Foley JJ, Ellis C, Zeng Z, Su K, Jurewicz AJ, Hertzberg RP, Bergsma DJ, Kumar C (1996) Molecular cloning and characterization of the human anaphylatoxin C3a receptor. J Biol Chem 271:20231–20234

Barnum SR (1995) Complement biosynthesis in the central nervous system. Crit Rev Oral Biol Med 6:132–146

Barnum SR, Ames RS, Maycox PR, Hadingham SJ, Meakin J, Harrison D, Parsons AA (2002) Expression of the complement C3a and C5a receptors after permanent focal ischemia: An alternative interpretation. Glia 38:169–173

Bellander BM, von Holst H, Fredman P, Svensson M (1996) Activation of the complement cascade and increase of clusterin in the brain following a cortical contusion in the adult rat. J Neurosurg 85:468–475

Bellander BM, Singhrao SK, Ohlsson M, Mattsson P, Svensson M (2001) Complement activation in the human brain after traumatic head injury. J Neurotrauma 18:1295–1311

Botto M, Dell'Agnola C, Bygrave AE, Thompson EM, Cook HT, Petry F, Loos M, Pandolfi PP, Walport MJ (1998) Homozygous C1q deficiency causes glomerulonephritis associated with multiple apoptotic bodies. Nat Genet 19:56–59

Boulay F, Mery L, Tardif M, Brouchon L, Vignais P (1991) Expression cloning of a receptor for C5a anaphylatoxin on differentiated HL-60 cells. Biochemistry 30:2993–2999

Carney DF, Lang TJ, Shin ML (1990) Multiple signal messengers generated by terminal complement complexes and their role in terminal complement complex elimination. J Immunol 145:623–629

Crass T, Raffetseder U, Martin U, Grove M, Klos A, Kohl J, Bautsch W (1996) Expression cloning of the human C3a anaphylatoxin receptor (C3aR) from differentiated U-937 cells. Eur J Immunol 26:1944–1950

Czurko A, Nishino H (1994) Appearance of immunoglobulin G and complement factor C3 in the striatum after transient focal ischemia in the rat. Neurosci Lett 166:51–54

Daffern PJ, Pfeifer PH, Ember JA, Hugli TE (1995) C3a is a chemotaxin for human eosinophils but not for neutrophils I C3a stimulation of neutrophils is secondary to eosinophil activation. J Exp Med 181:2119–2127

Dandoy-Dron F, Guillo F, Benboudjema L, Deslys JP, Lasmezas C, Dormont D, Tovey MG, Dron M (1998) Gene expression in scrapie Cloning of a new scrapie-responsive gene and the identification of increased levels of seven other mRNA transcripts. J Biol Chem 273:7691–7697

del Zoppo GJ (1999) In stroke, complement will get you nowhere. Nat Med 5:995–996

De Simoni MG, Storini C, Barba M, Catapano L, Arabia AM, Rossi E, Bergamaschini L (2003) Neuroprotection by complement (C1) inhibitor in mouse transient brain ischemia. J Cereb Blood Flow Metab 23:232–239

Di Napoli M (2001) Systemic complement activation in ischemic stroke. Stroke 32:1443–1448

Dietzschold B, Schwaeble W, Schafer MK, Hooper DC, Zehng YM, Petry F, Sheng H, Fink T, Loos M, Koprowski H, et al (1995) Expression of C1q, a subcomponent of the rat complement system, is dramatically enhanced in brains of rats with either Borna disease or experimental allergic encephalomyelitis. J Neurol Sci 130:11–16

Ehlers MR (2000) CR3: a general purpose adhesion-recognition receptor essential for innate immunity. Microbes Infect 2:289–294

Ember JA, Hugli TE (1997) Complement factors and their receptors. Immunopharmacology 38:3–15

Ember JA, Jagels MA, Hugli TE (1998) Characterization of complement anaphylatoxins and biological responses. In: The Human Complement

System in Health and Disease JE Volanakis and MM Frank, editors Marcel Dekker, New York, NY p 241

Farkas I, Baranyi L, Takahashi M, Fukuda A, Liposits Z, Yamamoto T, Okada H (1998a) A neuronal C5a receptor and an associated apoptotic signal transduction pathway. J Physiol 507:679–687

Farkas I, Baranyi L, Liposits ZS, Yamamoto T, Okada H (1998b) Complement C5a anaphylatoxin fragment causes apoptosis in TGW neuroblastoma cells. Neuroscience 86:903–911

Fischer B, Schmoll H, Riederer P, Bauer J, Platt D, Popa-Wagner A (1995) Complement C1q and C3 mRNA expression in the frontal cortex of Alzheimer's patients. J Mol Med 73:465–471

Frank MM, Fries LF (1991) The role of complement in inflammation and phagocytosis. Immunol Today 12:322–326

Gasque P, Julen N, Ischenko AM, Picot C, Mauger C, Chauzy C, Ripoche J, Fontaine M (1992) Expression of complement components of the alternative pathway by glioma cell lines. J Immunol 149:1381–1387

Gasque P, Ischenko A, Legoedec J, Mauger C, Schouft MT, Fontaine M (1993) Expression of the complement classical pathway by human glioma in culture. A model for complement expression by nerve cells J Biol Chem 268:25068–25074

Gasque P, Fontaine M, Morgan BP (1995) Complement expression in human brain. Biosynthesis of terminal pathway components and regulators in human glial cells and cell lines. J Immunol 154:4726–4733

Gasque P, Thomas A, Fontaine M, Morgan BP (1996) Complement activation on human neuroblastoma cell lines in vitro: route of activation and expression of functional complement regulatory proteins. J Neuroimmunol 66:29–40

Gasque P, Dean YD, McGreal EP, van Beek J, Morgan BP (2000) Complement components of the innate immune system in health and disease in the CNS. Immunopharmacology 49:171–186

Gerard, NP, Gerard C (1991) The chemotactic receptor for human C5a anaphylatoxin. Nature 349:614–617

Guan E, Robinson SL, Goodman EB, Tenner AJ (1994) Cell-surface protein identified on phagocytic cells modulates the C1q-mediated enhancement of phagocytosis. J Immunol 152:4005–4016

Heese K, Hock C, Otten U (1998) Inflammatory signals induce neurotrophin expression in human microglial cells. J Neurochem 70:699–707

Huang J, Kim LJ, Mealey R, Marsh HC Jr, Zhang Y, Tenner AJ, Connolly ES Jr, Pinsky DJ (1999) Neuronal protection in stroke by an sLex-glycosylated complement inhibitory protein. Science 285:595–599

Imagawa DK, Osifchin NE, Paznekas WA, Shin ML, Mayer MM (1983) Consequences of cell membrane attack by complement: release of arachidonate and formation of inflammatory derivatives. Proc Natl Acad Sci USA 80:6647–6651

Kaczorowski SL, Schiding JK, Toth CA, Kochanek PM (1995) Effect of soluble complement receptor-1 on neutrophil accumulation after traumatic brain injury in rats. J Cereb Blood Flow Metab 15:860–864

Kasuya H, Shimizu T (1989) Activated complement components C3a and C4a in cerebrospinal fluid and plasma following subarachnoid hemorrhage. J Neurosurg 71:741–746

Kildsgaard J, Hollmann TJ, Matthews KW, Bian K, Murad F, Wetsel RA (2000) Cutting edge: targeted disruption of the C3a receptor gene demonstrates a novel protective anti-inflammatory role for C3a in endotoxin-shock. J Immunol 165:5406–5409

Krych-Goldberg M, Atkinson JP (2001) Structure-function relationships of complement receptor type 1. Immunol Rev 180:112–122

Levi-Strauss M, Mallat M (1987) Primary cultures of murine astrocytes produce C3 and factor B, two components of the alternative pathway of complement activation. J Immunol 139:2361–2366

Lindsberg PJ, Ohman J, Lehto T, Karjalainen-Lindsberg ML, Paetau A, Wuorimaa T, Carpen O, Kaste M, Meri S (1996) Complement activation in the central nervous system following blood–brain barrier damage in man. Ann Neurol 40:587–596

Martin U, Bock D, Arseniev L, Tornetta MA, Ames RS, Bautsch W, Kohl J, Ganser A, Klos A (1997) The human C3a receptor is expressed on neutrophils and monocytes, but not on B or T lymphocytes. J Exp Med 186:199–207

Mason JC, Yarwood H, Sugars K, Morgan BP, Davies KA, Haskard DO (1999) Induction of decay-accelerating factor by cytokines or the membrane-attack complex protects vascular endothelial cells against complement deposition. Blood 94:1673-1682

McGreal EP, Ikewaki N, Akatsu H, Morgan BP, Gasque P (2002) Human C1qRp is identical with CD93 and the mNI-11 antigen but does not bind C1q. J Immunol 168:5222–5232

Morgan BP (1989) Complement membrane attack on nucleated cells: resistance, recovery and non-lethal effects. Biochem J 264:1–14

Morgan BP (1996) Intervention in the complement system: a therapeutic strategy in inflammation. Biochem Soc Trans 24:224–229

Morgan BP, Gasque P (1996) Expression of complement in the brain: role in health and disease. Immunol Today 17:461–466

Morgan BP, Harris CL (1999) Complement Regulatory Proteins, eds BP Morgan and CL Harris Academic Press, San Diego

Mukherjee P, Pasinetti GM (2001) Complement anaphylatoxin C5a neuroprotects through mitogen-activated protein kinase-dependent inhibition of caspase 3. J Neurochem 77:43–49

Nataf S, Stahel PF, Davoust N, Barnum SR (1999) Complement anaphylatoxin receptors on neurons: new tricks for old receptors? Trends Neurosci 22:397–402

Niculescu F, Rus H, Shin S, Lang T, Shin ML (1993) Generation of diacylglycerol and ceramide during homologous complement activation. J Immunol 150:214–224

Osaka H, McGinty A, Hoepken UE, Lu B, Gerard C, Pasinetti GM (1999a) Expression of C5a receptor in mouse brain: role in signal transduction and neurodegeneration. Neuroscience 88:1073–1082

Osaka H, Mukherjee P, Aisen PS, Pasinetti GM (1999b) Complement-derived anaphylatoxin C5a protects against glutamate-mediated neurotoxicity. J Cell Biochem 73:303–311

Pasinetti GM, Johnson SA, Rozovsky I, Lampert-Etchells M, Morgan DG, Gordon MN, Morgan TE, Willoughby D, Finch CE (1992) Complement C1qB and C4 mRNAs responses to lesioning in rat brain. Exp Neurol 118:117–125

Roglic A, Prossnitz ER, Cavanagh SL, Pan Z, Zou A, Ye RD (1996) cDNA cloning of a novel G protein-coupled receptor with a large extracellular loop structure. Biochim Biophys Acta 1305:39–43

Rus HG, Niculescu FI, Shin ML (2001) Role of the C5b-9 complement complex in cell cycle and apoptosis. Immunol Rev 180:49–55

Rus HG, Niculescu F, Shin ML (1996) Sublytic complement attack induces cell cycle in oligodendrocytes. J Immunol 156:4892–4900

Rus H, Niculescu F, Badea T, Shin ML (1997) Terminal complement complexes induce cell cycle entry in oligodendrocytes through mitogen activated protein kinase pathway. Immunopharmacology 38:177–187

Rus H, Weerth S, Soane L, Niculescu F, Rus V, Raine CS, Shin ML (2002) The effect of terminal complement complex on apoptosis gene expression in experimental autoimmune encephalomyelitis. Int Immunol 2:1248

Sayah S, Ischenko AM, Zhakhov A, Bonnard AS, Fontaine M (1999) Expression of cytokines by human astrocytomas following stimulation by C3a and C5a anaphylatoxins: specific increase in interleukin-6 mRNA expression. J Neurochem 72:2426–2436

Schafer MK, Schwaeble WJ, Post C, Salvati P, Calabresi M, Sim RB, Petry F, Loos M, Weihe E (2000) Complement C1q is dramatically up-regulated in brain microglia in response to transient global cerebral ischemia. J Immunol 164:5446–5452

Shen Y, Li R, McGeer EG, McGeer PL (1997) Neuronal expression of mRNAs for complement proteins of the classical pathway in Alzheimer brain. Brain Res 769:391–395

Shirazi Y, McMorris FA, Shin ML (1989) Arachidonic acid mobilization and phosphoinositide turnover by the terminal complement complex, C5b-9, in rat oligodendrocyte x C6 glioma cell hybrids. J Immunol 142:4385–4391

Shirazi Y, Imagawa DK, Shin ML (1987) Release of leukotriene B4 from sublethally injured oligodendrocytes by terminal complement complexes. J Neurochem 48:271–278

Singhrao SK, Neal JW, Rushmere NK, Morgan BP, Gasque P (1999a) Differential expression of individual complement regulators in the brain and choroid plexus. Lab Invest 79:1247–1259

Singhrao SK, Neal JW, Morgan BP, Gasque P (1999b) Increased complement biosynthesis by microglia and complement activation on neurons in Huntington's disease. Exp Neurol 159:362–376

Singhrao SK, Neal JW, Rushmere NK, Morgan BP, Gasque P (2000) Spontaneous classical pathway activation and deficiency of membrane regulators render human neurons susceptible to complement lysis. Am J Pathol 157:905–918

Soane L, Rus H, Niculescu F, Shin ML (1999) Inhibition of oligodendrocyte apoptosis by sublytic C5b-9 is associated with enhanced synthesis of bcl-2 and mediated by inhibition of caspase-3 activation. J Immunol 163:6132–6138

Stahel PF, Frei K, Fontana A, Eugster HP, Ault BH, Barnum SR (1997a) Evidence for intrathecal synthesis of alternative pathway complement activation proteins in experimental meningitis. Am J Pathol 151:897–904

Stahel PF, Kossmann T, Morganti-Kossmann MC, Hans VH, Barnum SR (1997b) Experimental diffuse axonal injury induces enhanced neuronal C5a receptor mRNA expression in rats. Brain Res Mol Brain Res 50:205–212

Stahel PF, Nadal D, Pfister HW, Paradisis PM, Barnum SR (1997c) Complement C3 and factor B cerebrospinal fluid concentrations in bacterial and aseptic meningitis. Lancet 349:1886–1887

Stahel PF, Kariya K, Shohami E, Barnum SR, Eugster H, Trentz O, Kossmann T, Morganti-Kossmann MC (2000) Intracerebral complement C5a receptor (CD88) expression is regulated by TNF and lymphotoxin-alpha following closed head injury in mice. J Neuroimmunol 109:164–172

Stahel PF, Morganti-Kossmann MC, Perez D, Redaelli C, Gloor B, Trentz O, Kossmann (2001) Intrathecal levels of complement-derived soluble membrane attack complex (sC5b-9) correlate with blood–brain barrier dysfunction in patients with traumatic brain injury. J Neurotrauma 18:773–781

Sunyer JO T, Zarkadis IK, Lambris JD (1998) Complement diversity: a mechanism for generating immune diversity? Immunol Today 19:519–523

Taylor PR, Carugati A, Fadok VA, Cook HT, Andrews M, Carroll MC, Savill JS, Henson PM, Botto M, Walport MJ (2000) A hierarchical role for classical pathway complement proteins in the clearance of apoptotic cells in vivo. J Exp Med 192:359–366

Thomas A, Gasque P, Vaudry D, Gonzalez B, Fontaine M (2000) Expression of a complete and functional complement system by human neuronal cells in vitro. Int Immunol 12:1015–1023

van Beek J, Chan P, Bernaudin M, Petit E, MacKenzie ET, Fontaine M (2000a) Glial responses, clusterin, and complement in permanent focal cerebral ischemia in the mouse. Glia 31:39–50 van Beek J, Bernaudin M, Petit E, Gasque P, Nouvelot A, MacKenzie ET, Fontaine M (2000b) Expression of receptors for complement anaphylatoxins C3a and C5a following permanent focal cerebral ischemia in the mouse. Exp Neurol 161:373–382

van Beek J, Nicole O, Ali C, Ischenko A, MacKenzie ET, Buisson A, Fontaine M (2001) Complement anaphylatoxin C3a is selectively protective against NMDA-induced neuronal cell death. Neuroreport 12:289–293

Vasthare US, Barone FC, Sarau HM, Rosenwasser RH, DiMartino M, Young WF, Tuma RF (1998) Complement depletion improves neurological function in cerebral ischemia. Brain Res Bull 45:413–419

Walker DG, McGeer PL (1992) Complement gene expression in human brain: comparison between normal and Alzheimer disease cases. Brain Res Mol Brain Res 14:109–116

Wetsel RA (1995) Structure, function and cellular expression of complement anaphylatoxin receptors. Curr Opin Immunol 7:48–53

Wiedmer T, Ando B, Sims PJ (1987) Complement C5b-9-stimulated platelet secretion is associated with a Ca2+-initiated activation of cellular protein kinases. J Biol Chem 262:13674–13681

Witte DP, Welch TR, Beischel LS (1991) Detection and cellular localization of human C4 gene expression in the renal tubular epithelial cells and other extrahepatic epithelial sources. Am J Pathol 139:717–724

Xiong ZQ, Qian W, Suzuki K, McNamara JO (2003) Formation of complement membrane attack complex in mammalian cerebral cortex evokes seizures and neurodegeneration. J Neurosci 23:955–960

Yasojima K, McGeer EG, McGeer PL (1999a) Complement regulators C1 inhibitor and CD59 do not significantly inhibit complement activation in Alzheimer disease. Brain Res 833:297–301

Yasojima K, Schwab C, McGeer EG, McGeer PL (1999b) Up-regulated production and activation of the complement system in Alzheimer's disease brain. Am J Pathol 154:927–936

Zwirner J, Fayyazi A, Gotze O (1999) Expression of the anaphylatoxin C5a receptor in non-myeloid cells. Mol Immunol 36:877–884

Zwirner J, Gotze O, Begemann G, Kapp A, Kirchhoff K, Werfel T (1999) Evaluation of C3a receptor expression on human leucocytes by the use of novel monoclonal antibodies. Immunol 97:166–172

5 Inflammation in Stroke: The Good, the Bad, and the Unknown

U. Dirnagl

It has been known for a very long time (Spielmeyer 1922) that in 'apoplectic' brains the hallmarks of inflammation may be found, including pus-filled cavities. Until very recently it was generally believed that brain inflammation following stroke is a secondary reaction to the destruction of brain tissue, which is cleared by invading leukocytes, in particular macrophages (Manoonkitiwongsa et al. 2001). Accordingly, inflammation is supposed to free the brain from the debris of dead cells, but in itself does not participate in ischemic cell damage. Quite clearly, this concept must be modified in view of recent research. Numerous experimental as well as clinical studies have linked stroke-induced brain inflammation to the acute and delayed evolution of brain infarction, as well as to scattered selective neuronal injury in the infarct perimeter. These studies have been reviewed (e.g., Barone and Feuerstein 1999; del Zoppo et al. 2000,

2001; Kumar 2001; Iadecola and Alexander 2001; Emsley and Tyrrell 2002; Frijns and Kappelle 2002; Danton and Dietrich 2003) and
we wrote an overview entitled 'Inflammation in Stroke – A Potential
Target for Neuroprotection' (Priller and Dirnagl 2002) for the 2001
Ernst Schering Foundation Workshop 'Neuroinflammation – From
Bench to Bedside.' The accompanying chapters by the symposium
participants will summarize in depth what is known about brain inflammation and stroke. I would like to provide a very general frame-
work for generating and testing hypotheses concerning the prospects
of targeting inflammation in stroke. As will become apparent, the
matter is quite complex, and such interventions could be envisioned
to either inhibit or foster certain forms of inflammation. To avoid
confusion it should be stated here that while this review and the
Schering Symposium concentrate on inflammation induced by
stroke, the opposite phenomenon, that is, stroke induced by inflammation (Emsley and Tyrrell 2002; Gorelick 2002; Muir 2002; Paganini-Hill et al. 2003), although the subject of intense study and of
great clinical relevance for the prevention of stroke, does not lie
within the focus of our workshop and will therefore not be covered.
Likewise, the increased susceptibility after stroke to systemic inflammation and infection (Prass et al. 2003), which is of great importance for stroke outcome (already 24 h after a stroke infection is the
major cause of death in stroke patients; Grau et al. 1999; Langhorne
et al. 2000) will not be considered here.

5.1 The Problem

Stroke is the third leading cause of death in civilized countries, and
the most important cause of adult disabilities. In Germany alone
there are more than 200,000 new stroke cases every year; one-third
of these patients die acutely, one-third remain with severe disabilities, and only one-third recover with acceptable outcome. Thus,
from a public health perspective stroke is one of the most relevant
diseases, particularly since therapeutic options still are highly disap-
pointing: Thrombolysis with recombinant tissue plasminogen activator (rtPA), the only therapy with proven efficacy in a major clinical
trial (The National Institute of Neurological Disorders and Stroke

rtPA Stroke Study Group 1995), is only effective within a 3-h time window, limiting its application to less than a few percent of patients with ischemic stroke. In other words, besides basic supportive therapy, at present more than 95% of strokes cannot be treated specifically (Caso and Hacke 2002; Broderick and Hacke 2002).

In parallel with the demonstration of the efficacy of rtPA treatment in many countries, the infrastructure of stroke care has improved tremendously. This process has taught us that further improvements in infrastructure will be very limited, and in particular that time intervals from symptom onset to treatment below 3 h can only benefit a very small fraction of patients. A recent WHO study has revealed that at present even the best available acute care for stroke patients (stroke unit, thrombolysis, etc.) can only marginally improve outcome (Heller et al. 2000). This situation has triggered a search for novel brain protective strategies, targeting delayed mechanisms of damage.

Delayed treatment only makes sense if there is progression of the lesion over an extended time period. Until rather recently it was commonly held that infarcts in stroke evolve in a few hours – so why treat a structural deficit that is already fixed? However, concomitantly with the demonstration of delayed mechanisms of damage in experimental stroke models (Dirnagl et al. 1999), it was shown in animal models of the disease that indeed there can be maturation of the infarct over more than 24 h (Rudin et al. 2001), and that selective neuronal damage evolves around the lesion core with an even more delayed time course (Nedergaard 1987; Garcia et al. 1993). Modern neuroimaging methods and their increasingly widespread use in clinical stroke studies have allowed the validation of these findings in humans (Pantano et al. 1999). It is now accepted that in at least 30% of unselected patients with ischemic stroke, a progression of the lesion can be demonstrated on magnetic resonance (MR) or computed tomography (CT) images beyond 24 h after stroke onset.

5.2 Delayed Mechanisms of Damage –
Rodent Versus Human

What mechanisms might cause delayed lesion growth? There are numerous possibilities – which might be active alone or in combination: Progression of the vascular occlusion (e.g., by growth of the thrombus, or by further microembolization); ongoing excitotoxicity around the lesion core (e.g., periinfarct depolarizations, elevated excitatory amino acids, and depolarizing ions in general); programmed cell death (i.e., apoptosis); and last but not least inflammation. We should also not forget that there are primarily extracranial factors which may negatively affect the lesion, such as fever (which is common after stroke); normo- or even hypotension in previously hypertensive patients (which may be the result of therapy!), elevated blood glucose, etc., all of which are in the focus of basic care at stroke units.

In animals experiments most of these factors are tightly controlled (temperature, blood pressure, glucose, and oxygenation), and reperfusion is often induced (which stops periinfarct depolarizations almost immediately), and the thrombus cannot grow in most models (because not a thrombus but a filament occluded the intracranial vessel!). Thus, animal experiments may (over)emphazise the relative contribution of inflammation and apoptosis to delayed lesion growth. This is what disease models are for: they provide us with experimental strategies to isolate and characterize certain pathophysiological entities. But when generalizing from mouse to man we should keep in mind these differences. What this means is that we need independent evidence derived directly from clinical studies that inflammation is indeed a relevant mechanism in human stroke. Ideally, to cope with the tremendous variability in human stroke we need markers helping us to separate patients with ongoing inflammation from those without. If no inflammation is detected, the patient would be spared from therapy (which always has a risk of side effects). In addition, efficacy studies are more likely to show a beneficial effect if a rather homogenous study population is chosen where the targeted mechanism is actually present, and the 'dilution' of the treatment effect is minimized by the absence of the target.

Another issue here concerns age, and its effect on inflammation. Most animal experiments are carried out in adolescent rodents, while the typical stroke patient is senescent. It is well known that immune responses change with age (Gavazzi and Krause 2002; Castle 2000). In general, while there is no decrease in the number of immune cells with aging, their function changes. For example, there is an involution of the thymus and impairment of T-cell proliferation, and Th1 responses are decreased whereas Th2 responses are increased. Whether these immune changes are linked to the differences in infarct volume (Sutherland et al. 1996; Davis et al. 1995) and cavitation of experimental infarcts (Popa-Wagner et al. 1998) in old versus young animals is unknown, but differences in inflammation between old and young rodents have been described (Fotheringham et al. 2000; Siren et al. 1993; Liu et al. 1994). Clearly, further systematic study is needed to investigate the effect of aging on the extent and time course of inflammation in experimental stroke.

5.3 How to Detect Ongoing Stroke-Induced Brain Inflammation in Human

Presently, in stroke patients we can apply only rather indirect approaches to search for inflammation in the brain. Blood plasma is of course available for screening of soluble markers of inflammation, which may be derived from the activated brain endothelium in the inflamed region, or may have diffused from the brain parenchyma into the blood and cerebrospinal fluid (CSF), which can also be collected and screened. Markers that have been used thus far include soluble ICAM-1, IL-1, TNF, and CRP, among others (Love and Barber 2001; Zaremba and Losy 2001, 2002; Di Napoli 2001; Frijns and Kappelle 2002; Marquardt et al. 2002; Tanne et al. 2002). Blood leukocytes, which may have had contact with activated brain endothelium or even patrolled the brain (like, e.g., lymphocytes) may have become activated themselves, which can be assayed (Elneihoum et al. 1996). Leukocytes and inflammatory proteins that have entered the CSF are another indicator for an inflammatory process in the brain parenchyma (Suzuki et al. 1995; Kostulas et al. 1999). However, all these markers suffer from various drawbacks, most importantly a complete lack of spatial resolution (where is the inflammation and what is its extent?), but also a rather ill-defined temporal resolution: inflammatory markers may be present in the blood or CSF at a time when the process in the brain parenchyma is no longer active or biologically relevant.

A promising approach to circumvent these limitations might be the molecular imaging of brain inflammation (Lewin et al. 2000; Weissleder et al. 2000; Louie et al. 2000; Bremer et al. 2001; Lok 2001; Becker et al. 2001; Ntziachristos et al. 2002; Chen et al. 2002; Weissleder and Ntziachristos 2003). One hallmark of brain inflammation is the upregulation of endothelial adhesion molecules, guiding white blood cells to the brain parenchyma. With the use of proper ligands (e.g., peptide-antibodies raised against adhesion molecules) coupled to dyes for optical detection in the near-infrared wavelength range (e.g., indocyanine dyes), or to radiochemicals for positron emission tomography (PET) detection, or to MR-contrast agents (e.g., MION particles), brain inflammation could be noninvasively localized and quantified. While proof of principle experiments demonstrating the feasibility of molecular imaging of brain pathophysiology with PET, optical, and MR methodologies have been successfully carried out in animal experiments, the challenge now is the adaptation of molecular imaging to human stroke.

5.4 Inflammation – Friend or Foe?

A host of articles link inflammation in stroke to the progression of damage. The pillars of the 'perpetrator' dogma on the negative effects of stroke induced inflammation are:

1. Inflammation/inflammatory cells can be found in brain after stroke
2. Anti-inflammatory strategies protect against experimental stroke
3. Animals with targeted disruption of genes linked to inflammation (iNOS, COX2, etc.) are protected against stroke
4. Inflammatory markers are present in the serum and CSF of stroke patients and correlate with outcome
5. Inducing brain inflammation/inflammatory mediators causes brain damage

Thus, inhibition of inflammation would seem to be a straightforward therapeutic strategy. However, inflammation is a relevant strategy of any tissue to cope not only with the invasion of pathogens, but also with tissue destruction (Wyss-Coray and Mucke 2002). Inflammation plays an important part in the clearing of destroyed tissue, and in the following process of angiogenesis, tissue remodeling, and regeneration (Moore 1999; Lingen 2001). This is probably best studied in wound healing, which is severely compromised if inflammation is inhibited or disrupted by gene targeting (Gallucci et al. 2000). The potential benefits of inflammation after stroke have received relatively little attention thus far, but indirect evidence suggests that certain types of inflammatory reactions are neuroprotective and neuroregenerative, which will be the topic of some of the accompanying chapters, in particular those of Hallenbeck and Schwartz (Chaps. 7 and 8, respectively). In brief, macrophages and microglia produce a host of trophic cytokines when activated, and macrophages or T cells exposed to certain CNS antigens ex vivo partake in tissue repair and recovery after nerve transsection and spinal cord injury (Neumann 2000; Schwartz 2001).

Despite the existence of numerous articles linking inflammation (in particular brain influx of leukocytes) with brain damage in stroke, some caution should be exerted. A recent review has reevaluated the available evidence for a pathogenic role of leukocytes in stroke (Emerich et al. 2002). Upon testing the available literature against the principles of (1) temporal ordering, (2) dose escalation, (3) topographic relationship, and (4) modulatory neuroprotection, Emerich et al. concluded that the available literature 'consistently falls short of establishing a clear cause–effect relationship between leukocyte recruitment and the pathogenesis of ischemia.'

It is very likely that tissue destruction or protection by inflammation is critically influenced by the degree of activation of inflammatory cells, their cellular identity, and timing. One hypothesis is that early on after stroke (i.e., the first hours and days), highly activated inflammatory cells (such as neutrophils and macrophages) contribute to the expansion of the lesion, while at later time points mildly activated glial cells and subsets of T lymphocytes exert protective and regenerative effects. Since the discrimination between (putative) protective and destructive effects of inflammation has a great impact on therapeutic strategies (When should we treat? Which inflammatory mechanism should be targeted?), this issue should be clarified in experimental models before such strategies are translated into clinical medicine.

5.5 The Ideal Target

Ideally, the target for (anti)inflammatory therapy should play a relevant role in tissue destruction after stroke, be active long enough to present a favorable therapeutic window, be upstream in inflammatory signaling cascades so that interference with it has broad effects on downstream effectors of damage, be accessible to drugs given intravenously, and play no major role in the healthy brain (and body, if targeted i.v.), among other desirable features. At present it appears that inflammatory enzymes such as inducible nitric oxide synthase (iNOS), cyclooxygenase-2 (COX-2), and endothelial adhesion molecules (such as ICAM-1) fulfill at least some of these criteria. Less well studied, but nevertheless very attractive, are strategies which prime and instruct the adaptive immune system to brain protective responses (see accompanying chapters by Schwartz and Hallenbeck; Takeda et al. 2002; Nevo et al. 2003).

5.6 The Ideal Drug

The ideal drug, on the other hand, should affect the inflammatory mechanism(s) selectively, get access to the site of action via the i.v. route, and have a favorable safety profile and pharmacokinetics. From the viewpoint of a rapid translation from bench to bedside it may also be desirable to choose a drug that has a longstanding history in the treatment of other diseases (as, e.g., COX-2 inhibitors in rheumatoid arthritis). This approach, however, is very often not compatible with the search by the pharmaceutical industry for novel and proprietary drugs which can be commercially exploited for a relevant time period.

5.7 Where Do We Go From Here?

Are we ready to treat human stroke as an 'ischemia-induced ence-phalitis'? The experimental evidence for a relevant contribution of inflammatory mechanisms to delayed tissue damage in stroke is very strong. Several targets appear very promising, in particular some endothelial or leukocyte adhesion molecules, and key enzymes of inflammatory free radical production. In addition, for some of these targets promising drugs are already available, some newly developed, proprietary ones, as well as some well established, safe compounds currently used for different indications. However, several stroke trials testing anti-inflammatory approaches have so far failed (see accompanying chapter by del Zoppo, Chap. 9), and no large clinical trials (http://www.strokecenter.org) targeting inflammation in stroke appear to be currently under way. In the future, strategies which direct and instruct the inflammatory machinery may turn out to be superior to the suppression of inflammation.

Given the difficulties in translating basic science to the bedside, we should not hasten the application of strategies targeting inflammation in human stroke, and we should learn from the experience provided by the largely unsuccessful clinical stroke trials targeting excitotoxicity (Kidwell et al. 2001). At the bench we need to better understand how we can selectively block the destructive mechanisms of inflammation after stroke, and possibly even foster potential protective ones. This involves a deeper understanding of stroke-induced 'encephalitis', and of regeneration and plasticity of the brain after injury in general. At the bedside we need to develop tools to noninvasively monitor and quantify brain inflammation after injury, and to design better clinical trials with enough statistical power to demonstrate a potential benefit of these novel strategies.

At present, treatment of stroke patients is very limited. Targeting inflammation after stroke appears to have great potential. This potential should be explored with great care by basic researchers and clinicians alike.

Acknowledgements. The author's work is supported by the Hermann and Lilly Schilling Foundation and the Deutsche Forschungsgemeinschaft.

References

Barone FC, Feuerstein GZ (1999) Inflammatory mediators and stroke: new opportunities for novel therapeutics. J Cereb Blood Flow Metab 19:819–834

Becker A, Hessenius C, Licha K, Ebert B, Sukowski U, Semmler W, Wiedenmann B, Grotzinger C (2001) Receptor-targeted optical imaging of tumors with near-infrared fluorescent ligands. Nat Biotechnol 19:327–331

Bremer C, Tung CH, Weissleder R (2001) In vivo molecular target assessment of matrix metalloproteinase inhibition. Nat Med 7:743–748

Broderick JP, Hacke W (2002) Treatment of acute ischemic stroke: Part I: recanalization strategies. Circulation 106:1563–1569

Caso V, Hacke W (2002) The very acute stroke treatment: fibrinolysis and after. Clin Exp Hypertens 24:595–602

Castle SC (2000) Clinical relevance of age-related immune dysfunction. Clin Infect Dis 31:578–85.

Chen J, Tung CH, Mahmood U, Ntziachristos V, Gyurko R, Fishman MC, Huang PL, Weissleder R (2002) In vivo imaging of proteolytic activity in atherosclerosis. Circulation 105:2766–2771

Danton GH, Dietrich WD (2003) Inflammatory mechanisms after ischemia and stroke. J Neuropathol Exp Neurol 62:127–136

Davis M, Mendelow AD, Perry RH, Chambers IR, James OF (1995) Experimental stroke and neuroprotection in the aging rat brain. Stroke 26:1072–8.

del Zoppo G, Ginis I, Hallenbeck JM, Iadecola C, Wang X, Feuerstein GZ (2000) Inflammation and stroke: putative role for cytokines, adhesion molecules and iNOS in brain response to ischemia. Brain Pathol 10:95–112

del Zoppo GJ, Becker KJ, Hallenbeck JM (2001) Inflammation after stroke: is it harmful? Arch Neurol 58:669–672

Di Napoli M (2001) Early inflammatory response in ischemic stroke. Thromb Res 103:261–264

Dirnagl U, Iadecola C, Moskowitz MA (1999) Pathobiology of ischaemic stroke: an integrated view. Trends Neurosci 22:391–397

Elneihoum AM, Falke P, Axelsson L, Lundberg E, Lindgarde F, Ohlsson K (1996) Leukocyte activation detected by increased plasma levels of inflammatory mediators in patients with ischemic cerebrovascular diseases. Stroke 27:1734–1738

Emerich DF, Dean RL 3rd, Bartus RT (2002) The role of leukocytes following cerebral ischemia: pathogenic variable or bystander reaction to emerging infarct? Exp Neurol 173:168–81.

Emsley HC, Tyrrell PJ (2002) Inflammation and infection in clinical stroke. J Cereb Blood Flow Metab 22:1399–1419

Fotheringham AP, Davies CA, Davies I. (2000) Oedema and glial cell involvement in the aged mouse brain after permanent focal ischaemia. Neuropathol Appl Neurobiol 26:412–23.

Frijns CJ, Kappelle LJ (2002) Inflammatory cell adhesion molecules in ischemic cerebrovascular disease. Stroke 33:2115–2122

Gallucci RM, Simeonova PP, Matheson JM, Kommineni C, Guriel JL, Sugawara T, Luster MI (2000) Impaired cutaneous wound healing in interleukin-6-deficient and immunosuppressed mice. FASEB J 14:2525–2531

Garcia JH, Yoshida Y, Chen H, Li Y, Zhang ZG, Lian J, Chen S, Chopp M (1993) Progression from ischemic injury to infarct following middle cerebral artery occlusion in the rat. Am J Pathol 142:623–635

Gavazzi G, Krause KH (2002) Ageing and infection. Lancet Infect Dis 2:659–66

Gorelick PB (2002) Stroke prevention therapy beyond antithrombotics: unifying mechanisms in ischemic stroke pathogenesis and implications for therapy: an invited review. Stroke 33:862–875

Grau AJ, Buggle F, Schnitzler P, Spiel M, Lichy C, Hacke W (1999) Fever and infection early after ischemic stroke. J Neurol Sci 171:115–120

Heller RF, Langhorne P, James E (2000) Improving stroke outcome: the benefits of increasing availability of technology. Bull World Health Organ 78:1337–43

Iadecola C, Alexander M (2001) Cerebral ischemia and inflammation. Curr Opin Neurol 14:89–94

Kidwell CS, Liebeskind DS, Starkman S, Saver JL (2001) Trends in acute ischemic stroke trials through the 20th century. Stroke 32:1349–1359

Kostulas N, Pelidou SH, Kivisakk P, Kostulas V, Link H (1999) Increased IL-1beta, IL-8, and IL-17 mRNA expression in blood mononuclear cells observed in a prospective ischemic stroke study. Stroke 30:2174–2179

Kumar K (2001) Overview: pro-inflammatory cytokines in cerebrovascular ischemia. Curr Opin Investig Drugs 2:1748–1750

Langhorne P, Stott DJ, Robertson L, MacDonald J, Jones L, McAlpine C, Dick F, Taylor GS, Murray G (2000) Medical complications after stroke: a multicenter study. Stroke 31:1223–1229

Lewin M, Carlesso N, Tung CH, Tang XW, Cory D, Scadden DT, Weissleder R (2000) Tat peptide-derivatized magnetic nanoparticles allow in vivo tracking and recovery of progenitor cells. Nat Biotechnol 18:410–414

Lingen MW (2001) Role of leukocytes and endothelial cells in the development of angiogenesis in inflammation and wound healing. Arch Pathol Lab Med 125:67–71

Liu Y, Jacobowitz DM, Barone F, McCarron R, Spatz M, Feuerstein G, Hallenbeck JM, Siren AL (1994) Quantitation of perivascular monocytes and
   macrophages around cerebral blood vessels of hypertensive and aged
   rats. J Cereb Blood Flow Metab 14:348–52

Lok C (2001) Picture perfect. Nature 412:372–374

Louie AY, Huber MM, Ahrens ET, Rothbacher U, Moats R, Jacobs RE, Fra-
   ser SE, Meade TJ (2000) In vivo visualization of gene expression using
   magnetic resonance imaging. Nat Biotechnol 18:321–325

Love S, Barber R (2001) Expression of P-selectin and intercellular adhesion
   molecule-1 in human brain after focal infarction or cardiac arrest. Neuropathol Appl Neurobiol 27:465–473

Manoonkitiwongsa PS, Jackson-Friedman C, McMillan PJ, Schultz RL, Lyden PD (2001) Angiogenesis after stroke is correlated with increased
   numbers of macrophages: the clean-up hypothesis. J Cereb Blood Flow
   Metab 21:1223–1231

Marquardt L, Ruf A, Mansmann U, Winter R, Schuler M, Buggle F, Mayer
   H, Grau AJ (2002) Course of platelet activation markers after ischemic
   stroke. Stroke 33:2570–2574

Moore K (1999) Cell biology of chronic wounds: the role of inflammation.
   J Wound Care 8:345–348

Muir KW (2002) Inflammation, blood pressure, and stroke: an opportunity
   to target primary prevention? Stroke 33:2732–2733

Nedergaard M (1987) Neuronal injury in the infarct border: a neuropathological study in the rat. Acta Neuropathol (Berl) 73:267–274

Neumann H (2000) The immunological microenvironment in the CNS: implications on neuronal cell death and survival. J Neural Transm Suppl
   59:59–68

Nevo U, Kipnis J, Golding I, Shaked I, Neumann A, Akselrod S, Schwartz
   M (2003) Autoimmunity as a special case of immunity: removing threats
   from within. Trends Mol Med 9:88–93

Ntziachristos V, Tung CH, Bremer C, Weissleder R (2002) Fluorescence molecular tomography resolves protease activity in vivo. Nat Med 8:757–
   760

Paganini-Hill A, Lozano E, Fischberg G, Perez BM, Rajamani K, Ameriso
   SF, Heseltine PN, Fisher M (2003) Infection and risk of ischemic stroke:
   differences among stroke subtypes. Stroke 34:452–457

Pantano P, Caramia F, Bozzao L, Dieler C, von Kummer R (1999) Delayed
   increase in infarct volume after cerebral ischemia: correlations with
   thrombolytic treatment and clinical outcome. Stroke 30:502–507

Popa-Wagner A, Schroder E, Walker LC, Kessler C (1998) beta-Amyloid
   precursor protein and ss-amyloid peptide immunoreactivity in the rat
   brain after middle cerebral artery occlusion: effect of age. Stroke
   29:2196–202.

Prass K, Meisel D, Hoflich C, Braun J, Halle E, Wolf T, Ruscher K, Victo-
   rov IV, Priller J, Dirnagl U, Volk HD, Meisel A (2003) Stroke-induced

immunodeficiency promotes spontaneous bacterial infections and is mediated by sympathetic activation – reversal by post-stroke Th1-like immunostimulation. J Exp Med 198:735–736

Priller J, Dirnagl U (2002) Inflammation in stroke – a potential target for neuroprotection? Ernst Schering Res Found Workshop 133–157

Rudin M, Baumann D, Ekatodramis D, Stirnimann R, McAllister KH, Sauter A (2001) MRI analysis of the changes in apparent water diffusion coefficient, T(2) relaxation time, and cerebral blood flow and volume in the temporal evolution of cerebral infarction following permanent middle cerebral artery occlusion in rats. Exp Neurol 169:56–63

Schwartz M (2001) T cell mediated neuroprotection is a physiological response to central nervous system insults. J Mol Med 78:594–597

Siren AL, Liu Y, Feuerstein G, Hallenbeck JM (1993) Increased release of tumor necrosis factor-alpha into the cerebrospinal fluid and peripheral circulation of aged rats. Stroke 24:880–6

Spielmeyer W (1922) Allgemeine Histopathologie des Nervensystems. (in German), Springer, Berlin, Germany

Sutherland GR, Dix GA, Auer RN (1996) Effect of age in rodent models of focal and forebrain ischemia. Stroke 27:1663–7

Suzuki S, Kelley RE, Reyes-Iglesias Y, Alfonso VM, Dietrich WD (1995) Cerebrospinal fluid and peripheral white blood cell response to acute cerebral ischemia. South Med J 88:819–824

Takeda H, Spatz M, Ruetzler C, McCarron R, Becker K, Hallenbeck J (2002) Induction of mucosal tolerance to E-selectin prevents ischemic and hemorrhagic stroke in spontaneously hypertensive genetically stroke-prone rats. Stroke 33:2156–63

Tanne D, Haim M, Boyko V, Goldbourt U, Reshef T, Matetzky S, Adler Y, Mekori YA, Behar S (2002) Soluble intercellular adhesion molecule-1 and risk of future ischemic stroke: a nested case-control study from the Bezafibrate Infarction Prevention (BIP) study cohort. Stroke 33:2182–2186

The National Institute of Neurological Disorders and Stroke rt-PA Stroke Study Group (1995) Tissue plasminogen activator for acute ischemic stroke. N Engl J Med 333:1581–1587

Weissleder R, Moore A, Mahmood U, Bhorade R, Benveniste H, Chiocca EA, Basilion JP (2000) In vivo magnetic resonance imaging of transgene expression. Nat Med 6:351–355

Weissleder R, Ntziachristos V (2003) Shedding light onto live molecular targets. Nat Med 9:123–128

Wyss-Coray T, Mucke L (2002) Inflammation in neurodegenerative disease–a double-edged sword. Neuron 35:419–432

Zaremba J, Losy J (2001) Early TNF-alpha levels correlate with ischaemic stroke severity. Acta Neurol Scand 104:288–295

Zaremba J, Losy J (2002) sPECAM-1 in serum and CSF of acute ischaemic stroke patients. Acta Neurol Scand 106:292–298

6 Tetracycline Derivatives as Anti-inflammatory Agents and Potential Agents in Stroke Treatment

J. Koistinaho, J. Yrjänheikki, T. Kauppinen, M. Koistinaho

6.1 Introduction

Tetracyclines are well-known bacteriostatic drugs with a broad-spectrum antimicrobial activity. The first tetracycline was isolated more than 50 years ago, reaching the market in 1953. The widely used semisynthetic tetracycline derivatives, doxycycline and minocycline (Fig. 1), were synthesized in 1966 and 1972, respectively (Sande and Mandel 1985). Today, minocycline is the most widely prescribed systemic antibiotic for acne, and in the UK alone, over 6.5 million people receive long-term treatment (9 months in average) with it. The antibiotic resistance is low with minocycline compared with

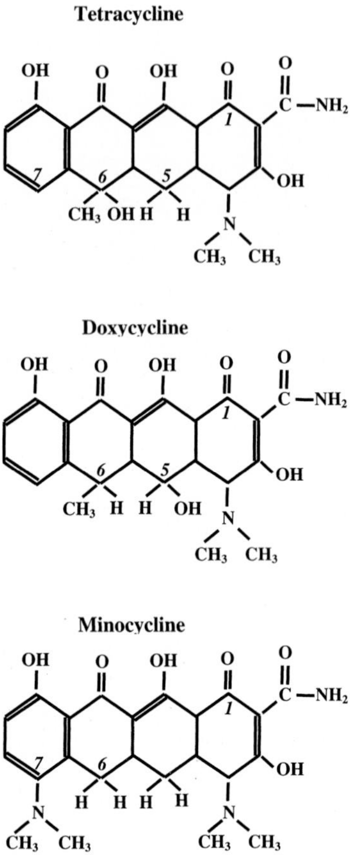

Fig. 1. The molecular structure of tetracycline and its semisynthetic derivatives, minocycline and doxycycline. Note the differences in substitute groups of carbons 6 and 7 in minocycline and of carbons 5 and 6 in doxycycline

other tetracyclines and antibiotics. In general, minocycline is considered a safe drug in humans. Severe drug reactions include drug-induced lupus, hypersensitivity syndrome reaction, and serum sickness-like reaction, but there are only 1.6 cases per million exposures, making these adverse reactions very rare.

In 1984 Golub and colleagues reported that minocycline and some other tetracyclines inhibit collagenase (matrix metalloprotease) activity. After this initial finding on non-antimicrobial mechanisms of action for tetracycline derivatives, minocycline was found to depress oxygen radical release from polymorphonuclear neutrophils (Gabler and Creamer 1991; Gabler et al. 1992), inhibit inducible nitric oxide synthase (Amin et al. 1996), and scavenge superoxide (van Barr et al. 1987) and peroxynitrate (Whiteman and Halliwell 1997). Because inflammation is thought to contribute to ischemic stroke, and minocycline has a superior tissue penetration into the brain, in 1996 we initiated a research program to investigate whether minocycline could be a potential therapeutic drug for treatment of stroke. Here we review our results on different animal and cell culture models of ischemic brain injury.

6.2 Minocycline in a Global Ischemia Model

Transient, severe global ischemia arising in humans as a consequence of cardiac arrest or cardiac surgery or induced experimentally in animals leads to selective and delayed neuronal death, particularly of pyramidal neurons in the hippocampal CA1 (Choi 1996). Global ischemia-induced neuronal death is not detected until 3–5 days after induction of global ischemia in rats and gerbils. The relative contributions of apoptotic and necrotic death to ischemia-induced neuronal loss remain controversial (MacManus and Buchan 2000; Yamashima 2000), but microgliosis (Gehrmann et al. 1992) and induction of pro-inflammatory genes, such as cyclooxygenase-2 (Koistinaho et al. 1999) and inducible nitric oxide synthase (iNOS) (Endoh et al. 1994) are known to occur and may contribute to the neuronal injury after global brain ischemia.

Using global gerbil ischemia as a model, we first screened the effect of three different tetracyclines: tetracycline, doxycycline, and minocycline. We also included two other broadly used antibiotics, erythromycin and ceftriaxone, as these two drugs had previously been found to be neuroprotective in cell culture models (Rothstein and Kuncl 1995). The antibiotics were administered intraperitoneally twice a day starting 24 h before ischemia, and the treatment was continued until the day the animals were sacrificed (Yrjänheikki et al. 1998). The screening studies indicated neuroprotective potential of only doxycycline and minocycline, which together with tetracycline were studied more in detail in the same gerbil model. We used the dose of 180–90 mg/kg per day because the treatment did not result in severe side effects and the maximal penetration of the drugs to the brain was desired. Twelve hours before ischemia, gerbils were injected with 45 mg/kg of minocycline, doxycycline, or tetracycline hydrochloride. Thereafter, the animals were injected twice a day, at a dose of 90 mg/kg during the first day after ischemia and 45 mg/kg starting 36 h after ischemia. The postischemic treatment was started 30 min after ischemia with 90 mg/kg. Both the minocycline and doxycycline treatments significantly increased the number of surviving neurons. Six days after ischemia, the minocycline-pretreated gerbils had 76.7%, minocycline-posttreated gerbils had 71.4%, doxycycline-pretreated gerbils had 57.2%, and doxycycline-posttreated gerbils had 47.1% of the neuron profiles left in the CA1 pyramidal cell layer, whereas in untreated gerbils 10.5% of the CA1 neurons were left. The neuroprotection was statistically significant in every animal group. Tetracycline did not provide any protection. Minocycline and doxycycline did not reduce the postoperative body temperatures.

To determine whether neuroprotection by minocycline is associated with activation of nonneuronal cells, we studied GFAP expression, a marker of astrogliosis, and phosphotyrosine immunoreactivity and isolectin B4 binding, which are markers of activated microglia. The results showed that expression of GFAP mRNA in the hippocampus was increased to the same extent in saline- and minocycline-treated gerbils and that immunoreactivity for GFAP was similar in these two groups. Instead, microglial activation appeared to be significantly reduced in minocycline-treated gerbils. We therefore next studied whether induction of interleukin 1β-converting enzyme (ICE), an apoptosis-promoting gene that is strongly induced in microglia after global ischemia, or iNOS, an enzyme suggested to produce toxic concentration of nitric oxide in nonneuronal cells after global brain ischemia (Endoh et al. 1994), are affected by neuroprotective minocycline treatment. The semiquantitative RT-PCR showed that 4 days after ischemia, expression of ICE mRNA was attenuated by approximately 70% and expression of iNOS mRNA by 30% in the hippocampus of minocycline-treated gerbils. In addition, 6 days after ischemia, NADPH-diaphorase-reactive cells were seen in the hippocampi of saline-treated, but not in minocycline-treated, ischemic gerbils. Most of the NADPH-diaphorase-reactive cells resembling microglia were located in the pyramidal cell layer of the CA1 subfield, and some NADPH-diaphorase-reactive cells with the morphology typical of astrocytes were detected in the stratum radiatum. Therefore, minocycline inhibited NOS activity also in astrocytes, even though it did not block astrogliosis.

Altogether, the studies on the global ischemia model indicated that minocycline and doxycycline protect against global brain ischemia even when administered after the ischemic insult. Importantly, minocycline reduced expression of proinflammatory genes, ICE and iNOS, and prevented microgliosis, suggesting that inflammation plays a role in ischemia-induced death of hippocampal neurons.

6.3 Minocycline in a Focal Ischemia Model

6.3.1 Transient Ischemia Models

Because minocycline was more neuroprotective than doxycycline in global brain ischemia, we decided to continue with minocycline in a transient focal brain ischemia model of the rat (Yrjänheikki et al. 1999). Treatment with minocycline (45 mg/kg i.p. twice a day for the first day; 22.5 mg/kg for the subsequent 2 days) did not affect rectal temperature, arterial blood pressure, plasma glucose, or arterial blood gases. However, the treatment started 12 h before 90-min ischemia reduced the size of the infarct in the cerebral cortex by 76% and in the striatum by 39%. Starting the minocycline treatment 2 h after the onset of ischemia resulted in a reduction in the size of cortical (by 65%) and striatal (by 42%) infarct, a reduction similar to the one obtained with pretreatment. The cortical infarct size was reduced by 63% even when the treatment was started 4 h after the onset of ischemia.

Because cortical spreading depression (SD), an energy-consuming wave of transient depolarizations of astrocytes and neurons, contributes to the evolution of ischemia to infarction in focal ischemia

(Mies et al. 1993; Back et al. 1996; Busch et al. 1996), we tested whether minocycline provides protection by inhibiting cortical SD. In a separate set of rats that were not subjected to middle cerebral artery occlusion (MCAO), minocycline did not alter the number, duration, or amplitude of direct current potentials induced by a 60-min exposure to topical 3 M KCl, whereas MK-801, an NMDA receptor antagonist known to reduce partially ischemic damage by blocking cortical SD, completely prevented KCl-induced direct current potentials. Thus, this experiment excluded inhibition of SD as a mechanism of action for minocycline.

As nonneuronal cells are characteristically activated in the brain in response to ischemic injury (Banati et al. 1993; Giulian and Corpuz 1993; McGeer and McGeer 1995), and minocycline was found to reduce microglial activation in a global ischemia model, we studied astrogliosis and microglial activation in a focal ischemia model. At 24 h after 90 min of ischemia, a strong induction of CD11b immunoreactivity was observed around and inside the infarction core in untreated rats. The immunoreactive cells had an amoeboid shape in the penumbra zone. Minocycline treatment started 12 h before ischemia decreased the number of CD11b-immunoreactive cells and prevented the appearance of the amoeboid-shaped microglia adjacent to the infarction core. Instead, GFAP immunoreactivity in the ischemic hemispheres of untreated and minocycline-treated animals was similarly increased. Similar to global ischemia studies, pretreatment with minocycline also decreased the induced ICE mRNA levels by 83% in the penumbra, indicating that minocycline treatment inhibits expression of the enzyme needed for interleukin (IL)-1β activation in microglia.

COX-2 is highly expressed in the brain after global and focal brain ischemia and produces superoxides and proinflammatory prostaglandins such as PGE_2 (Sairanen et al. 1998; Nogawa et al. 1997; Miettinen et al. 1997; Koistinaho et al. 1999). In general, expression of COX-2 is reduced by anti-inflammatories and can be induced by cytokines, including IL-1β. Because minocycline treatment inhibited microglial activation, we studied whether the treatment also affects COX-2. In global brain ischemia of gerbil, we studied the hippocampal expression of COX-2 mRNA and found that minocycline downregulated the expression by 30%–40%. The protein levels and activity of COX-2 were studied in a focal brain ischemia model. In untreated rats, the PGE_2 concentration was increased fivefold in the ischemic penumbra and was preceded by the induction of COX-2-immunoreactive neurons. Pretreatment with minocycline reduced the PGE_2 concentration in the penumbra by 55% and almost completely prevented the appearance of COX-2 immunoreactivity at 24 h.

6.3.2 Permanent Ischemia Model

Given that minocycline rescues brain tissue in transient focal ischemia with a wide therapeutic window but that a majority of MCAOs in humans is not associated with reperfusion during the first hours, the next experiments were directed to test whether minocycline and doxycycline also protect against permanent ischemia (Koistinaho et al. 2003). For this purpose we used several mouse lines to exclude the possibility that the possible protection is strain-dependent. Minocycline and doxycycline were injected at 12-h intervals at the dose of 60 mg/kg during the first 24 h after the ischemia and thereafter at the dose of 45 mg/kg until sacrifice. The mice were subjected to 24-h or 72-h permanent MCAO, and the infarction injuries were analyzed histologically using TTC staining or by T2-weighted magnetic resonance imaging. Again, minocycline did not alter physiological variables such as body temperature, blood gases or pH, or plasma glucose. When the treatment was started 12 h prior to the onset of ischemia, the infarct volume was reduced in FVB/N mice by 33% at 24 h. To study the effect of minocycline and doxycycline in longer treatment protocols, Balb/C mice were exposed to 72-h permanent ischemia. Aminoguanidine, administered 200 mg/kg at 12-h intervals beginning 24 h after the onset of MCAO, was used as a positive control. We found that minocycline reduced the infarction volumes by 28% and doxycycline by 25% compared to saline-treated control mice. As expected, aminoguanidine treatment also provided significant (−33%) protection. However, when minocycline treatment was started 2 h after the insult, only a 10% reduction, which was not significant, was detected in the infarction volumes. These results suggest that tetracycline derivatives may be beneficial only when perfusion occurs within few hours after the onset of ischemia. Alternatively, tetracyclines could serve as preventive therapies for stroke.

6.4 Mechanism Studies on Cell Culture Models

Tetracyclines, including minocycline, efficiently reduce inflammation in the peripheral system, for example by inhibiting the function of polymorphonuclear neutrophils (Gabler and Creamer 1991; Gabler et al. 1992) and the activity of matrix metalloproteases (MMP) (Golub et al. 1984; Paemen et al. 1996). To determine whether minocycline has direct effects on the brain cells, we studied minocycline in primary neuronal cultures (Tikka and Koistinaho 2001; Tikka et al. 2001 a,b; 2002) which were exposed to glutamic acid, kainic acid, and N-methyl-D-aspartate (NMDA), three excitotoxins thought to be involved in brain ischemia (Dirnagl et al. 1999). Mixed spinal cord cultures consisting of neurons (70%), astrocytes (24%), and microglia (6%) and devoid of endothelial cells and peripheral cells were used. When the cultures were exposed to 500 µM glutamate or 100 µM kainic acid for 24 h, or challenged for 5 min with 300 µM NMDA stimulus that was followed by 24 h incubation, we found that about 40%–60% of the neurons died. Importantly, administration of minocycline 30 min before the excitotoxin exposure reduced neuronal death dose-dependently. The maximal neuroprotection was achieved by 2–20 µM minocycline. We also observed that the neuronal death triggered by glutamate or kainic acid occurred at least partially through apoptosis, which was inhibited by minocycline as detected by nuclear binding bis-benzamide stain and DNA laddering. On the other hand, neuronal death induced by NMDA occurred through necrosis. Thus, minocycline protects against excitotoxicity by inhibiting both apoptotic and necrotic cell death.

6.4.1 Activation of Microglia in Excitotoxicity

We found that in our cell culture model the excitotic cell death was coupled with a two- to threefold increase in the number of ox-42 immunoreactive microglia (Tikka and Koistinaho 2001; Tikka et al. 2001 a). Even the sublethal doses of excitotoxins were able to increase the number of microglial cells. In addition, the release of IL-1β, a cytokine released mainly by microglia, was increased. To investigate whether the microglial proliferation in response to excitotoxicity is secondary to neuronal death, we exposed neuron-free mixed glial cultures to 500 μM concentrations of the three excitotoxins and found that the proliferation of microglia was not dependent on the presence of neurons. Most importantly, when pure primary microglia cultures were exposed to the excitotoxins, a two- to fourfold microglial proliferation was triggered as detected by 5-bromo-2-deoxyuridine (BrdU) staining. In addition, a four- to fivefold increase in nitric oxide and two- to threefold increase in IL-1β release was observed as a sign of microglial activation. These results suggested that excitoxins activate microglia by a mechanism that does not involve neuronal death.

To test the hypothesis that excitotoxin-induced microglial activation and proliferation precede neuronal death, we compared the time course of the changes in OX-42-positive cells and LDH release during a 24-h follow-up period. We found that the number of OX-42-IR cells was significantly increased already after 12 h, whereas the LDH release was increased significantly only after 24 h after exposure to 500 μM glutamate or 100 μM kainic acid. This result indicated that microglial proliferation and/or CD11b surface antigen expression starts prior to the onset of neuronal death. The finding led to the notion that increasing the number of microglial cells present in the neuronal cell culture could enhance the excitotoxic cell death. To test this idea, we cultured pure microglial cells on top of spinal cord cell cultures, which resulted in a threefold increase in the proportion of these cells. Both basal LDH release and the excitotoxin-induced LDH release were significantly enhanced within 24 h in these microglia-enriched cultures compared to normal spinal cord cultures, indicating that microglial activation is potentially detrimental to neurons and that it enhances excitotoxic neuronal death.

6.4.2 Minocycline Inhibits Excitotoxicity by Blocking p38 MAPK in Microglia

Numerous studies have demonstrated that mitogen-activated protein kinases (MAPKs) are involved in microglial activation and neuronal death. Thus, we studied whether a 10-min exposure to glutamic acid (500 μM), kainic acid (100 μM), or NMDA (300 μM) would cause alteration in phospho-p38 and phospho-p44/42 MAPK immunoreactivity in our neuronal cultures. We found that the activated, phosphorylated form of p38 MAPK was detected only in microglial cells (Tikka and Koistinaho 2001; Tikka et al. 2001a). Moreover, the number of p38 MAPK immunoreactive microglial cells was increased after excitotoxic insult, and this response was inhibited by adding minocycline to the cultures 30 min before the exposure. To confirm the role of p38 MAPK in minocycline-mediated neuroprotection, we tested the effect of SB203580, a specific p38 MAPK inhibitor, and PD98059, a specific p44/42 MAPK inhibitor. According to LDH release measured 24 h after the insult, inhibition of p38 MAPK, but not p44/42 MAPK, significantly reduced the excitotoxic neuronal death.

Finally, in pure microglial cultures, glutamate stimulation induced transiently a significant elevation of phospho-p38 MAPK, and this upregulation was downregulated by treatment with 200 nM minocycline.

Altogether, our findings indicated that one of the neuroprotective mechanisms of minocycline is inhibition of p38 MAPK in microglia, thereby preventing activation of these cells and the release of harmful neurotoxins and inflammatory cytokines.

6.5 Potential Mechanisms of Minocycline's Neuroprotection

Minocycline was recently tested in models of various brain diseases. In these studies, minocycline was found to be protective in neurodegenerative diseases such as Parkinson's disease (Du et al. 2001; He et al. 2001; Wu et al. 2002; Lin et al. 2003), Huntington's disease (Chen et al. 2000), multiple sclerosis (Popovic et al. 2002; Brundula et al. 2002; Zhang et al. 2003), and amyotrophic lateral sclerosis (Kriz et al. 2002; Tikka et al. 2002; van den Bosch et al. 2002; Zhang et al. 2003; Zhu et al. 2002). In addition, minocycline has been confirmed to be beneficial in acute brain injuries, including brain trauma (Sanchez Mejia et al. 2001), hypoxic-ischemic injury (Arvin et al. 2002), and embolic stroke (Wang et al. 2003). Whether minocycline represents an effective therapeutic in humans will be

Table 1. Proposed therapeutic targets for tetracycline derivatives

Proposed target of tetracyclines	References
MMP9 activity	Golub et al. 1984; Paemen et al. 1996; Brundula et al. 2002
MMP9 expression	Brundula et al. 2002; Koistinaho et al. 2003
Microglial activation	Yrjänheikki et al. 1998, 1999; Tikka et al. 2001 a, b, c, 2002; Kriz et al. 2002; Wu et al. 2002
p38 MAPK activity	Tikka et al. 2001 a, b; Kriz et al. 2002; Du et al. 2002; Lin et al. 2001
iNOS expression	Amin et al. 1996; Yrjänheikki et al. 1998; Sanchez Meija et al. 2000; Wu et al. 2002
ICE/caspase expression/ activity	Yrjänheikki et al. 1998, 1999; Sanchez Meija et al. 2000; Chen et al. 2000
COX-2 expression	Yrjänheikki et al. 1999
Cytochrome c release	Zhu et al. 2002
ROS production	Akamatsu et al. 1991; Lin et al. 2003
Superoxide/peroxinitrate scavenge	van Barr et al. 1987; Whiteman and Halliwell 1997
PLA$_2$	Pruzanski et al. 1998
Leukocyte functions	Brundula et al. 2002; Gabler and Creamer 1991

first tested in clinical trials of amyotrophic lateral sclerosis and Huntington's disease, which are currently in progress. A case study supporting the beneficial role of minocycline in Huntington's disease has been published (Denovan-Wright et al. 2002).

As a result of the recent minocycline studies, new potential mechanisms of action have been revealed for minocycline (Table 1). It is conceivable that while minocycline and other tetracycline derivatives may have several targets in the nervous system, the key direct targets of this drug may still remain to be discovered.

Acknowledgements. Our studies were supported by the Sigrid Juselius Foundation, Finland.

References

Akamatsu H, Niwa Y, Kurokawa I, Masuda R, Nishijima S, Asada Y (1991) Effects of subminimal inhibitory concentrations of minocycline on neutrophil chemotactic factor production in comedonal bacteria, neutrophil phagocytosis and oxygen metabolism. Arch Dermatol Res 283:524–528

Amin AR, Attur MG, Thakker GD, Patel PD, Vyas PR, Patel RN, Patel IR, Abramson SB (1996) A novel mechanism of action of tetracyclines: effects on nitric oxide synthases. Proc Natl Acad Sci USA 93:14014–14019

Arvin KL, Han BH, Du Y, Lin SZ, Paul SM, Holtzman DM (2002) Minocycline markedly protects the neonatal brain against hypoxic-ischemic injury. Ann Neurol 52:54–61

Back T, Ginsberg MD, Dietrich WD, Watson BD (1996) Induction of spreading depression in the ischemic hemisphere following experimental middle cerebral artery occlusion: effect on infarct morphology. J Cereb Blood Flow Metab 16:202–213

Banati RB, Gehrmann J, Schubert P, Kreutzberg GW (1993) Cytotoxicity of microglia. Glia 7:111–118

Brundula V, Rewcastle NB, Metz LM, Bernard CC, Yong VW (2002) Targeting leukocyte MMPs and transmigration: minocycline as a potential therapy for multiple sclerosis. Brain 125:1297–1308

Busch E, Gyngell ML, Eis M, Hoehn-Berlage M, Hossmann KA (1996) Potassium-induced cortical spreading depressions during focal cerebral ischemia in rats: contribution to lesion growth assessed by diffusion-weighted NMR and biochemical imaging. J Cereb Blood Flow Metab 16:1090–1099

Chen M, Ona VO, Li M, Ferrante RJ, Fink KB, Zhu S, Bian J, Guo L, Farrell LA, Hersch SM, Hobbs W, Vonsattel JP, Cha JH, Friedlander RM (2000) Minocycline inhibits caspase-1 and caspase-3 expression and delays mortality in a transgenic mouse model of Huntington disease. Nat Med 6:797–801

Choi DW (1996) Ischemia-induced neuronal apoptosis. Curr Opin Neurobiol 6:667–672

Denovan-Wright EM, Devarajan S, Dursun SM, Robertson HA (2002) Maintained improvement with minocycline of a patient with advanced Huntington's disease. J Psychopharmacol 16:393–394

Dirnagl U, Iadecola C, Moskowitz MA (1999) Pathobiology of ischaemic stroke: an integrated view. Trends Neurosci 22:391–397

Du Y, Ma Z, Lin S, Dodel RC, Gao F, Bales KR, Triarhou LC, Chernet E, Perry KW, Nelson DL, Luecke S, Phebus LA, Bymaster FP, Paul SM (2001) Minocycline prevents nigrostriatal dopaminergic neurodegeneration in the MPTP model of Parkinson's disease. Proc Natl Acad Sci USA 98:14669–14674

Endoh M, Maiese K, Wagner J (1994) Expression of the inducible form of nitric oxide synthase by reactive astrocytes after transient global ischemia. Brain Res 651:92–100

Gabler WL, Creamer HR (1991) Suppression of human neutrophil functions by tetracyclines. J Periodontal Res 26:52–58

Gabler WL, Smith J, Tsukuda N (1992) Comparison of doxycycline and a chemically modified tetracycline inhibition of leukocyte functions. Res Commun Chem Pathol Pharmacol 78:151–160

Gehrmann J, Bonnekoh P, Miyazawa T, Oschlies U, Dux E, Hossmann KA, Kreutzberg GW (1992) The microglial reaction in the rat hippocampus following global ischemia: immuno-electron microscopy. Acta Neuropathol (Berl) 84:588–595

Giulian D, Corpuz M (1993) Microglial secretion products and their impact on the nervous system. Adv Neurol 59:315–320

Golub LM, Ramamurthy N, McNamara TF, Gomes B, Wolff M, Casino A, Kapoor A, Zambon J, Ciancio S, Schneir M, et al. (1984) Tetracyclines inhibit tissue collagenase activity. A new mechanism in the treatment of periodontal disease. J Periodontal Res 19:651–655

He Y, Appel S, Le W (2001) Minocycline inhibits microglial activation and protects nigral cells after 6-hydroxydopamine injection into mouse striatum. Brain Res 909:187–193

Koistinaho J, Koponen S, Chan PH (1999) Expression of cyclooxygenase-2 mRNA after global ischemia is regulated by AMPA receptors and glucocorticoids. Stroke 30:1900–1905

Koistinaho M, Lappetelainen T, Kettunen M, Kauppinen RA, Opdenakker G, Koistinaho J (2003) The protective effect of minocycline in permanent ischemia is matrix metalloprotease-9 dependent. Submitted.

Kriz J, Nguyen MD, Julien JP (2002) Minocycline slows disease progression in a mouse model of amyotrophic lateral sclerosis. Neurobiol Dis 10: 268–278

Lin S, Zhang Y, Dodel R, Farlow MR, Paul SM, Du Y (2001) Minocycline blocks nitric oxide-induced neurotoxicity by inhibition p38 MAP kinase in rat cerebellar granule neurons. Neurosci Lett 315:61–64

Lin S, Wei X, Xu Y, Yan C, Dodel R, Zhang Y, Liu J, Klaunig JE, Farlow M, Du Y (2003) Minocycline blocks 6-hydroxydopamine-induced neurotoxicity and free radical production in rat cerebellar granule neurons. Life Sci 72:1635–1641

MacManus JP, Buchan AM (2000) Apoptosis after experimental stroke: fact or fashion? J Neurotrauma 17:899–914

McGeer PL, McGeer EG (1995) The inflammatory response system of brain: implications for therapy of Alzheimer and other neurodegenerative diseases. Brain Res Rev 21:195–218

Mies G, Iijima T, Hossmann KA (1993) Correlation between peri-infarct DC shifts and ischaemic neuronal damage in rat. Neuroreport 4:709–711

Miettinen S, Fusco FR, Yrjänheikki J, Keinänen, R, Hirvonen T, Roivainen R, Närhi M, Hökfelt T, Koistinaho J (1997) Spreading depression and focal brain ischemia induce cyclooxygenase-2 in cortical neurons through N-methyl-D-aspartic acid-receptors and phospholipase A2. Proc Natl Acad Sci USA 94:6500–6505

Nogawa S, Zhang F, Ross ME, Iadecola C (1997) Cyclo-oxygenase-2 gene expression in neurons contributes to ischemic brain damage. J Neurosci 17:2746–2755

Paemen L, Martens E, Norga K, Masure S, Roets E, Hoogmartens J, Opdenakker G (1996) The gelatinase inhibitory activity of tetracyclines and chemically modified tetracycline analogues as measured by a novel microtiter assay for inhibitors. Biochem Pharmacol 52:105–111

Popovic N, Schubart A, Goetz BD, Zhang SC, Linington C, Duncan ID (2002) Inhibition of autoimmune encephalomyelitis by a tetracycline. Ann Neurol 51:215–223

Pruzanski W, Stefanski E, Vadas P, McNamara TF, Ramamurthy N, Golub LM (1998) Chemically modified non-antimicrobial tetracyclines inhibit activity of phospholipases A2. J Rheumatol 25:1807–1812

Rothstein JD, Kuncl RW (1995) Neuroprotective strategies in a model of chronic glutamate-mediated motor neuron toxicity. J Neurochem 65:643–651

Sairanen T, Ristimaki A, Karjalainen-Lindsberg ML, Paetau A, Kaste M, Lindsberg P (1998) Cyclooxygenase-2 is induced globally in infarcted human brain. Ann Neurol 43:738–747

Sanchez Mejia RO, Ona VO, Li M, Friedlander RM (2001) Minocycline reduces traumatic brain injury-mediated caspase-1 activation, tissue damage, and neurological dysfunction. Neurosurgery 48:1393–1399

Sande MA, Mandell GL (1985) Antimicrobial agents. In: Goodman LS, Gilman A (eds) The pharmacological basis of therapeutics. Macmillan, New York, pp 1170–1198

Tikka TM, Koistinaho JE (2001) Minocycline provides neuroprotection against N-methyl-D-aspartate neurotoxicity by inhibiting microglia. J Immunol 166:7527–7533

Tikka T, Fiebich BL, Goldsteins G, Keinanen R, Koistinaho J (2001a) Minocycline, a tetracycline derivative, is neuroprotective against excitotoxicity by inhibiting activation and proliferation of microglia. J Neurosci 21:2580–2588

Tikka T, Usenius T, Tenhunen M, Keinanen R, Koistinaho J (2001b) Tetracycline derivatives and ceftriaxone, a cephalosporin antibiotic, protect neurons against apoptosis induced by ionizing radiation. J Neurochem 78:1409–1414

Tikka TM, Vartiainen NE, Goldsteins G, Oja SS, Andersen PM, Marklund SL, Koistinaho J (2002) Minocycline prevents neurotoxicity induced by cerebrospinal fluid from patients with motor neurone disease. Brain 125:722–731

van Barr HM, van de Kerkhof PC, Mier PD, Happle R (1987) Tetracyclines are potent scavengers of the superoxide radical. Br J Dermatol 117:131–132

Van Den Bosch L, Tilkin P, Lemmens G, Robberecht W (2002) Minocycline delays disease onset and mortality in a transgenic model of ALS. Neuroreport 13:1067–1070

Whiteman M, Halliwell B (1997) Prevention of peroxynitrite-dependent tyrosine nitration and inactivation of alpha1-antiproteinase by antibiotics. Free Radic Res 26:49–56

Wang CX, Yang T, Shuaib A (2003) Effects of minocycline alone and in combination with mild hypothermia in embolic stroke. Brain Res 963:327–239

Wu DC, Jackson-Lewis V, Vila M, Tieu K, Teismann P, Vadseth C, Choi DK, Ischiropoulos H, Przedborski S (2002) Blockade of microglial activation is neuroprotective in the 1-methyl-4-phenyl-1,2,3,6-tetrahydropyridine mouse model of Parkinson disease. J Neurosci 22:1763–1771

Yamashima T (2000) Implication of cysteine proteases calpain, cathepsin and caspase in ischemic neuronal death of primates. Prog Neurobiol 62:273–295

Yrjanheikki J, Tikka T, Keinanen R, Goldsteins G, Chan PH, Koistinaho J (1999) A tetracycline derivative, minocycline, reduces inflammation and protects against focal cerebral ischemia with a wide therapeutic window. Proc Natl Acad Sci USA 96:13496–13500

Yrjanheikki J, Keinanen R, Pellikka M, Hokfelt T, Koistinaho J (1998) Tetracyclines inhibit microglial activation and are neuroprotective in global brain ischemia. Proc Natl Acad Sci USA 95:15769–15774

Zhang W, Narayanan M, Friedlander RM (2003) Additive neuroprotective effects of minocycline with creatine in a mouse model of ALS. Ann Neurol 53:267–270

Zhang SC, Goetz BD, Duncan ID (2003) Suppression of activated microglia promotes survival and function of transplanted oligodendroglial progenitors. Glia 41:191–198

Zhu S, Stavrovskaya IG, Drozda M, Kim BY, Ona V, Li M, Sarang S, Liu AS, Hartley DM, Wu du C, Gullans S, Ferrante RJ, Przedborski S, Kristal BS, Friedlander RM (2002) Minocycline inhibits cytochrome c release and delays progression of amyotrophic lateral sclerosis in mice. Nature 417:74–78

7 Induction of Mucosal Tolerance to E-Selectin Targets Immunomodulation to Activating Vessel Segments and Prevents Ischemic and Hemorrhagic Stroke

H. Takeda, M. Spatz, C. Ruetzler, R. McCarron, K. Becker,
J. Hallenbeck

7.1 Introduction

Inflammatory and immune reactions at blood vessel segments that lead to local release of proinflammatory cytokines and local activation of luminal endothelium can initiate stroke (Hallenbeck et al. 1988; Libby et al. 1995). These multipotent autocrine or paracrine mediators can regulate expression of leukocyte adhesion molecules, production of other cytokines, growth factors, and chemokines, and production of matrix metalloproteinases in atherosclerosis. Local endothelium integrates extracellular signals and cellular responses in different regions of the vascular tree (Rosenberg and Aird 1999). Scattered perivascular ring patterns of immunoreactive tumor necrosis factor-alpha (TNF-a), heme oxygenase-1 (HO-1), and manganese superoxide dismutase (MnSOD) within the brain parenchyma of normal rats reflect cyclic activation and inactivation of brain vessel segments (Ruetzler et al. 2001). These cycles appear to be more frequent and intense in stroke-prone animals. Stroke risk factors such as hypertension, diabetes, advanced age, and genetic predisposition to stroke can prepare rodent brain vessels for thrombosis and hemorrhage in response to a single provocative dose of bacterial lipopolysaccharide (LPS) that induces release of proinflammatory cytokines in a paradigm related to the local Shwartzman reaction (Hallenbeck et al. 1988; Siren et al. 2001). Conversion of the normally antithrombotic luminal surface of endothelial cells to a prothrombotic and proinflammatory state occurs in response to cytokines such as TNF-a, interleukin-1 (IL-1), and interferon gamma (IFN-γ), resulting in fibrin deposition and upregulation of adhesion molecules for platelets and leukocytes (Becker et al. 2000; McCarron et al. 1991; Pober and Cotran 1990).

We found in previous studies that controlling inflammation in the brain by inducing oral tolerance to the CNS antigen myelin basic protein (MBP) decreased infarct size after middle cerebral artery occlusion in the rat (Becker et al. 1997). Oral tolerance is a well-established model whereby through feeding of an antigen, immunologic tolerance is induced to that specific antigen (Weiner 1997). Orally administered antigen encounters the gut-associated lymphoid tissue (GALT), which forms a well-developed immune network. GALT evolved to protect the host from ingested pathogens, and, perhaps by necessity, developed the inherent property of preventing the host from reacting to ingested proteins. The schedule and amount of antigen feeding determines the mechanism of the tolerance. Clonal deletion of antigen-reactive T cells can occur after a single feeding of very high dose antigen (Chen et al. 1995); active tolerance with production of regulatory T cells occurs after repetitive feedings of low-dose antigen (Chen et al. 1994; Groux et al. 1997). Upon antigen restimulation, T cells that have been tolerized with a low-dose regimen secrete cytokines such as IL-10 and transforming growth factor $\beta 1$ (TGF-$\beta 1$), which suppress cell-mediated, or $T_H 1$, immune responses (Chen et al. 1994). Activation of these T cells is specific for the tolerizing antigen. However, the immunomodulatory cytokines secreted in response to activation have nonspecific effects. Thus, local immunosuppression will occur wherever the tolerizing antigen is present. This phenomenon, which is known as "active cellular regulation" or "bystander suppression", leads to relatively organ-specific immunosuppression (Faria and Weiner 1999). Other forms of mucosal tolerance have also been investigated, specifically the administration of antigen via the nasal or aerosol route. The nasal route appears equally efficient and, in some instances, even more effective than the oral route in suppressing autoimmune diseases in animal models (Metzler and Wraith 1996).

E-selectin is a cytokine-inducible glycoprotein that functions as a cell adhesion molecule and is largely restricted to endothelial cells. It mediates the adhesion of various leukocytes, including neutrophils, monocytes, eosinophils, natural killer (NK) cells, and a subset of T cells, to activated endothelium (Bevilacqua and Nelson 1993; Bevilacqua et al. 1989). The expression of E-selectin is induced on human endothelium in response to cytokines IL-1 and TNF-a through transcriptional upregulation (Montgomery et al. 1991). E-selectin becomes expressed on vascular endothelial tissue where vascular segments are becoming activated (Bevilacqua 1993).

Based on these data we tested the hypothesis that circulating lymphocytes tolerized by transmucosal administration of E-selectin could target activated vessel segments in the brain that express E-selectin. We postulated that these lymphocytes would then suppress the activation, prevent local thrombosis and hemorrhage, and, consequently, prevent stroke.

Non-booster group (single administration)

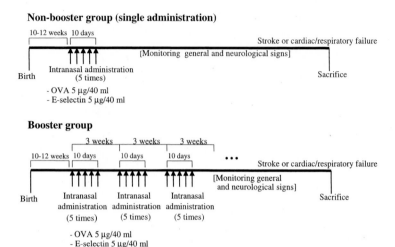

Fig. 1. Mucosal tolerization schedules

7.2 Repetitive Mucosal Tolerization to E-Selectin Prevents Ischemic and Hemorrhagic Stroke in Spontaneously Hypertensive, Genetically Stroke-Prone Rats

We administered ovalbumin or E-selectin to 10–12-week-old spontaneously hypertensive, genetically stroke-prone rats (SHR-SPs) as an intranasal instillation on a single or a repetitive course of tolerizations (Fig. 1). We examined the tolerized rats at least daily for the duration of their lives to detect signs of stroke (Yamori et al. 1982) or complications of severe hypertension such as cardiorespiratory failure associated with pulmonary edema. When signs of stroke or cardiorespiratory failure developed, we anesthetized the rats, collected blood samples and, after perfusion fixation, removed their brains for analysis. Despite the intensive monitoring, 10 of the 40 SHR-SPs initially divided among the four groups died between observations and were found unsuitable for further examination. We sectioned the remaining 30 perfused brains at eight predetermined stereotactic levels (Osborne et al. 1987) (240 sections), and stained them with hematoxylin-eosin for blinded quantification of the num-

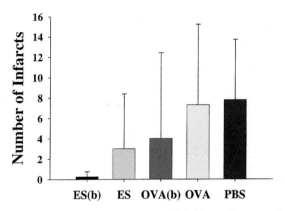

Fig. 2. Number of infarcts (mean±SD) per animal in each group. Groups on abscissa: *PBS*, phosphate buffered saline; *OVA*, ovalbumin; *OVA(b)*, ovalbumin booster; *ES*, E-selectin; *ES(b)*, E-selectin booster

bers and areas of infarcts (MetaMorph, Universal Imaging). The E-selectin single-course tolerization group (ES) had 12-fold more infarcts per animal than the E-selectin booster (ESb) group (3.00 vs. 0.25 averaged across the respective groups); corresponding stroke numbers for the ovalbumin booster (OVAb, 4.00) and ovalbumin single-course tolerization (OVA) groups (7.25) represented 16-fold and 29-fold increases, respectively, over ESb (Fig. 2). There were no hemorrhages in ESb, in contrast to 2.3, 3.2 and 2.8 hemorrhages per animal in ES, OVAb and OVA, respectively (Fig. 3). In order to utilize information on infarcts and/or hemorrhages with respect to the outcome of survival of the animals, we applied the Cox Proportional Hazard Model (Statistica). This nonparametric statistical method assumes that the underlying hazard rate (rather than survival time) is a function of other variables (covariates). Covariates were the number of infarcts and the number of intraparenchymal hemorrhages. For the number of infarcts, the analysis resulted in a chi-square=41.22, df=3, $P<0.00001$, and for the sum of the number of infarcts and the number of hemorrhages, the analysis resulted in a chi-square= 44.57, df=3, $P<0.00001$. Thus, for these two covariates, the four groups differ with respect to their hazard rate, i.e., the probability per time unit of failing in an interval given survival to the beginning

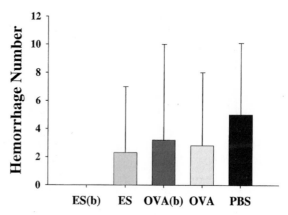

Fig. 3. Number of hemorrhages (mean+SD) per animal in each group. Groups are as defined in Fig. 2

of that interval. The average total areas of infarction and hemorrhage per animal totaled from the eight stereotactic sections were also lowest in ESb (0.002 mm^2, 0.0 mm^2, infarct and hemorrhage areas/animal, respectively) compared to ES (11.4 mm^2, 0.97 mm^2), OVAb (6.8 mm^2, 1.04 mm^2), and OVA (27.7 mm^2, 0.22 mm^2) groups; we were not able to perform stratified analyses of these covariates due to the limited data set. Lesions in affected animals were readily identifiable.

We subjected four additional animals to nasal instillation of phosphate buffered saline (PBS) and followed them until they developed stroke or cardiorespiratory failure. With respect to infarct number (7.8±5.9), infarct area (12.4±8.9 mm^2), and hemorrhage number (5.0±5.1), PBS closely resembled the OVA, OVAb, and ES group data listed above (Figs. 2, 3). Infarct area in PBS was highly variable and averaged 9.6±9.6 mm^2. Comparison of ESb and PBS (unpaired t-test) revealed significant differences in infarct number ($P < 0.004$), infarct area ($P < 0.002$), and hemorrhage number ($P < 0.02$).

Effective stroke prevention in the E-selectin booster group occurred despite persistent untreated hypertension. The initial and final blood pressures by the tail cuff method (that generally underestimates catheter-recorded values by at least 10 mmHg) were not different among the groups. The initial systolic blood pressures were (group mean±SD) 166±17 for ESb, 176±23 for ES, 164±8 for OVAb, and 174±21 for OVA. For the same four groups, the final systolic blood pressures were 192±26, 202±38, 189±22, and 211±36, respectively.

The animals lived for variable periods ranging from 14 weeks to the termination of the experiment at 56 weeks. Deaths were from heart failure secondary to severe hypertension as well as strokes. Differences in average age at time of death among the groups did not reach statistical significance. At the 56-week termination point, Kaplan-Meier survival curves estimated that 50% of ESb, 40% of the OVAb, and 30% of ES and OVA would survive the 56th week.

7.3 Mucosal Tolerization to E-Selectin Suppresses Delayed-Type Hypersensitivity

We demonstrated that intranasal instillation of human E-selectin does produce tolerance to a delayed-type hypersensitivity (DTH) paradigm described in Methods. The ear swelling in the group that received PBS tolerization before the sensitizing dose and subsequent challenge dose of E-selectin ($n=7$) was 0.36±0.18 mm (mean±SD) in comparison to the E-selectin tolerized group ($n=9$) 0.12±0.06 ($P<0.01$). Tolerance was antigen-specific since intranasal administration of OVA had no significant effect on DTH (results not shown).

7.4 Mucosal Tolerization to E-Selectin Produces Regulatory T Cells and Suppresses Vessel Activation

We harvested the spleen from 14-week-old SHR-SPs that had undergone a single-course tolerization with PBS, OVA, or E-selectin and intravenous injection of 0.45 mg/kg LPS two-weeks after tolerization to stimulate proinflammatory activation of blood vessels. Eight hours after LPS injection, we obtained 10 μm frozen spleen sections and stained for immunoreactive TGF-β. The E-selectin group had a significant increase in the number of TGF-β-positive cells, mainly in the periarteriolar lymphatic sheaths. TGF-β-positive cells colocalizing CD4, CD8, and ED2 (monocyte/macrophage) were present, but no single marker colocalized with a majority of positive cells. Serum levels of TGF-β after LPS injection did not differ among the groups. In addition, animals exposed to single-tolerization PBS, OVA, or ES produced detectible plasma IFN-γ in response to LPS (1,175±978, 827±959, 967±153 pg/ml, respectively, $n=3$–4); no IFN-γ response was observed in ES booster animals (3 tolerizations).

We instilled PBS, OVA, or E-selectin intranasally in 3–4 SHR-SPs per group on an initial tolerization schedule followed by two booster tolerizations. Two weeks after the second booster, we injected 0.45 mg/kg LPS to activate the vessel endothelium and processed the brains for ICAM-1 and E-selectin immunohistochemistry. ICAM-1 expression was significantly reduced in E-selectin-tolerized animals.

7.5 Antibody Formation

We did not detect anti-human E-selectin antibody in animals tolerized to E-selectin in either the stroke prevention or the DTH studies. In animals that received either single or repetitive E-selectin tolerization (three courses) followed 2 weeks later by intravenous LPS to activate endothelial expression of E-selectin, a detectible anti-human E-selectin antibody response did occur. Serum levels of anti-E-selectin antibodies were significantly elevated ($P<0.0001$) in animals tolerized by intranasal treatment with E-selectin as compared to PBS or OVA. The elevated levels of anti-E-selectin antibody seen in booster ES did not differ from those observed in single ES. Immunoreactive IgG anti-endothelial cell antibodies (AECAs) on luminal endothelium, however, were suppressed in single-tolerization E-selectin animals relative to ovalbumin and PBS single-tolerization animals that received LPS ($n=3$/group).

7.6 Discussion

The development of ischemic and hemorrhagic strokes in SHR-SP rats with untreated hypertension was potently inhibited by E-selectin booster tolerization. Tolerization to E-selectin also suppressed the delayed-type hypersensitivity response to that antigen. ESb animals exposed to intravenous LPS differed from animals in control groups; they had increased numbers of splenocytes positive for immunoreactive TGF-β, undetectable plasma levels of IFN-γ, and suppression of LPS-stimulated ICAM-1 expression on endothelium. In ESb, immunoreactive IgG binding to luminal endothelium was also suppressed. ES tolerization was not associated with formation of anti-E-selectin antibodies except in response to LPS stimulation.

The marked protection against thrombosis and hemorrhage in this study was antigen-specific and required that tolerization of lymphocytes be maintained as occurred in ESb. Vessel activation with E-selectin expression can therefore be inferred to precede the development of thrombosis or hemorrhage. Early stages in the development of thrombosis or hemorrhage can also be deduced to involve local inflammatory and immune mechanisms that can be aborted by tolerization of lymphocytes to a locally expressed antigen.

Support for the following model for the observed stroke prevention derives from our prior work (Ruetzler et al. 2001; Siren et al. 2001), studies of lymphocyte trafficking (von Andrian and Mackay 2000), and studies of the effector phase of mucosal tolerance (Faria and Weiner 1999; Miller et al. 1992). Circulating antigen-specific (tolerized) lymphocytes undergo a process of tethering, rolling, activation by chemokines, arrest with firm attachment, and diapedesis in vessel segments that have become activated by proinflammatory cytokines. Various adhesion molecules and paracrine signaling molecules mediate this process, and their assorted combinations guide selective migration of antigen-experienced cells to specific nonlymphoid tissues (Salmi et al. 1992). The initial steps in adhesion, tethering and rolling, are mediated by selectins and $\alpha 4\beta 1$ integrins. Chemokines, C5a (complement protein cleavage product), platelet activating factor, and leukotriene B4 are mediators of lymphocyte activation. Integrins on lymphocytes bind to endothelial immunoglobulin superfamily members to mediate arrest. Once arrested on an activated vessel segment or having migrated into vessel wall, antigen-specific lymphocytes can be re-stimulated. Antigen presentation through the trimolecular complex (MHC class II molecule, antigen, T-cell receptor) mediates re-stimulation. Endothelial cells that have been activated by IFN-γ (perhaps from CD4$^+$CD28^{null} NK-T cells (Liuzzo et al. 1999)) express MHC class II molecules and can serve as antigen-presenting cells (Hughes et al. 1990). Endocytosis of E-selectin expressed on vessels may facilitate presentation of that antigen (von Asmuth et al. 1992). Pericytes contact endothelial cells through fenestrations in the basal lamina, and along with perivascular macrophages can also serve as antigen-presenting cells in the vessel wall (Balabanov et al. 1999). Specific antigen presentation to T regulatory cells stimulates release of immunomodulatory cytokines such as TGF-β and/or IL-10 that provide active cellular regulation locally. These cytokines have broad immunosuppressive effects on lymphocytes and macrophages, inhibit inducible nitric oxide synthase, suppress superoxide anion generation, and reduce expression of E-selectin (Akdis and Blaser 2001; Prud'homme and Piccirillo 2000). The net effect decreases thrombogenicity and preserves vessel integrity.

The stroke prevention described in this report could be mediated by several alternative mechanisms. Although anti-E-selectin antibody was not detected in ESb; activation of endothelium with LPS did stimulate production of anti-E-selectin antibodies in ES-tolerized animals. The absence of anti-E-selectin antibody in ESb renders it unlikely that neutralizing anti-E-selectin antibodies prevented stroke by blocking that adhesion molecule in activated vessel segments (Zoldhelyi et al. 2000) of that group. Also due to functional redundancy with P-selectin (Labow et al. 1994), E-selectin$^{-/-}$ mice display no significant change in trafficking of leukocytes. Another possibility is that overall reduction of AECAs as shown by suppressed immunoreactive luminal IgG in ESb could have reduced local activation or apoptosis of endothelial cells (Bordron et al. 1998; George et al. 2000) and prevented strokes (Bordron et al. 2001). E-selectin tolerization may also have suppressed local activity of a functional T-cell subset associated with ischemia in unstable angina, IFN-γ-secreting CD4$^+$CD28^{null} NK-T cells (Weyand et al. 2001).

The overall effect of this intervention is to target immunosuppression to activated vessel segments. The precise molecular mecha-

nisms for the strong stroke prevention conferred by mucosal tolerization to E-selectin remain to be clarified, however. Evidence is accumulating that inflammatory and immune mechanisms can precipitate
cerebrovascular thrombosis and hemorrhage. Here we show that nasal instillation of E-selectin, a glycoprotein cell adhesion molecule
expressed specifically on activated endothelium, potently inhibits development of ischemic and hemorrhagic strokes in spontaneously hypertensive, genetically stroke-prone rats with untreated hypertension.
Repeated schedules of tolerization were required to maintain the resistance to stroke. Suppression of DTH to E-selectin and the presence of increased numbers of splenocytes positive for immunoreactive TGF-β showed that intranasal exposure to E-selectin induced
mucosal tolerance. E-selectin tolerization also reduced endothelial
activation in response to intravenous LPS, as shown by marked suppression of ICAM-1 expression compared to control animals. The
novel findings in this study support further investigation of immunological tolerance as applied to the prevention of stroke.

7.7 Methods

Male and female offspring of SHR-SP breeders were used (kind gift
of Professor Y. Yamori, Kyoto University, Japan) (10–12 weeks). Lit-
termates were distributed to maintain group blood pressure equiva-
lence. Intranasal instillations: (1) PBS (Bio-Whittaker), (2) ovalbumin, (albumin, chicken egg, grade V, Sigma), or (3) human E-selectin (lectin, EGF, CR1, CR2 domains, myc peptide tail kindly provided by Protein Design Labs).

7.7.1 Tolerization Schedule

Single (non-booster): PBS (20 µl), OVA (2.5 µg/20 µl), or E-selectin
(2.5 µg/20 µl) was instilled into each nostril every other day for
10 days (total of 5 administrations).

Repetitive (booster): intranasal instillations of the same substance
in the same volume and concentration on the same schedule as

above repeated at 3-week intervals for the lifetime of the animal or until the termination of the experiment.

7.7.2 Delayed-Type Hypersensitivity Reaction

A single-course tolerization schedule with either PBS or E-selectin was conducted ($n = 7,9$, respectively). Fourteen days later, animals were immunized (hind footpad) with 75 µg E-selectin/200 µl PBS plus 50 µl complete Freund's adjuvant (Sigma), the sensitizing dose. Fourteen days later, ear thickness was measured and the animals were rechallenged with 50 µg E-selectin/100 µl PBS injected into the ear, the challenge dose. Ear thickness increase over baseline was measured with microcalipers (Mitsutoyo) 2 days later.

7.7.3 Immunoassays

Commercial serum cytokine assays: OptEIA human TGF-β ELISA (PharMingen); Quantikine M rat IFN-γ immunoassay (R&D Systems).

ELISA plates (Nunc) coated overnight at 4 °C with 100 µl of 10 µg/ml recombinant human soluble E-selectin solution (sCD62E, R&D Systems, diluted to 10 µg/ml in coating buffer) in carbonate buffer, pH 9.5, blocked with 3% bovine serum albumin in PBS (2 h at RT). Plasma samples (100 µl/well) were added and plates incubated (2 h/RT). After washing, 100 µl biotinylated anti-rat F(ab')$_2$ IgG fragment (1:5,000 dilution) was added and plates incubated (2 h/RT); 100 µl 1:250 HRP-conjugated streptavidin were then added to each well. Wells were washed (×3 PBS/0.05% Tween-20) between each step, and plates were covered with adhesive strips during incubations. Anti-human E-selectin monoclonal antibody (biotin-conjugated mouse IgG1, clone #BBIG-E5, R&D Systems) confirmed plate coating and generated a standard curve. The standard curve generated for this assay was linear (0–100 ng/ml).

7.7.4 Immunofluorescence

Postfixed (acetone: methanol 1:1) spleen sections (10-μm) were stained for TGF-β as described (Barcellos-Hoff et al. 1995). Polyclonal anti-TGF-β, a kind gift from Kathy Flanders (NCI) was the primary; fluorescein-conjugated donkey anti-rabbit F(ab')$_2$ fragment (Jackson Immuno Research) was the detection antibody. Staining controls were omission of first antibody and substitution of rabbit IgG for primary antibody. Sections were analyzed for positive cells per visual field using an epifluorescence microscope (Axioplan, Carl Zeiss) with the appropriate filter. TGF-β-positive cells were double-stained with the following monoclonal antibodies: anti-rat CD4 (Cedarlane Laboratories), anti-rat CD8a (BDPharmingen), and anti-rat macrophages, Clone:ED2 (Biosource International).

7.7.5 Immunohistochemistry

Fresh frozen rat brain coronal sections (16-μm) were post-fixed with cold acetone (15 min) and stained for E-selectin or ICAM-1 as described (Okada et al. 1994). After blocking (5% normal donkey serum), antibody-binding sites were visualized (Vector ABC System, Vector Laboratories) using diaminobenzidine (DAB) as chromogen. Antibodies were: anti-rat E-selectin (1:500) (Protein Design Labs), anti-rat CD54 (1:100, Cedarlane), biotinylated donkey anti-mouse IgG F(ab')$_2$ (1:2000, Jackson Immuno Research). Sections were analyzed (Laborlux, Leitz) at ×100, and vessels expressing immunoreactivity for each antigen were counted in whole sections.

Immunoreactive IgG anti-AECAs were detected in frozen rat brain sections (16-μm) postfixed with cold acetone (15 min), blocked (5% normal donkey serum), and incubated overnight (4 °C) with (Fab')$_2$ biotinylated donkey anti-rat IgG (1:1000, Jackson Immuno Research). Antibody binding was visualized using the Vector ABC method with DAB. For quantitation of endothelial IgG expression, images (×100) of 10 cortical regions in both brain hemispheres were obtained (Axioplan, Zeiss) and analyzed (MetaMorph image processing system, Universal Imaging). IgG immunoreactivity was calculated as the percentage of visual field area positive for AECAs.

References

Akdis CA, Blaser K (2001) Mechanisms of interleukin-10-mediated immune suppression. Immunology 103:131–136

Balabanov R, Beaumont T, Dore-Duffy P (1999) Role of central nervous system microvascular pericytes in activation of antigen-primed splenic T-lymphocytes. J Neurosci Res 55:578–587

Barcellos-Hoff MH, Ehrhart EJ, Kalia M, Jirtle R, Flanders K, Tsang ML (1995) Immunohistochemical detection of active transforming growth factor-beta in situ using engineered tissue. Am J Pathol 147:1228–1237

Becker BF, Heindl B, Kupatt C, Zahler S (2000) Endothelial function and hemostasis. Z Kardiol 89:160–167

Becker KJ, McCarron RM, Ruetzler C, Laban O, Sternberg E, Flanders KC, Hallenbeck JM (1997) Immunologic tolerance to myelin basic protein decreases stroke size after transient focal cerebral ischemia. Proc Natl Acad Sci U S A 94:10873–10878

Bevilacqua MP (1993) Endothelial-leukocyte adhesion molecules. Annu Rev Immunol 11:767–804

Bevilacqua MP, Nelson RM (1993) Selectins. J Clin Invest 91:379–387

Bevilacqua MP, Stengelin S, Gimbrone MA, Jr, Seed B (1989) Endothelial leukocyte adhesion molecule 1: an inducible receptor for neutrophils related to complement regulatory proteins and lectins. Science 243:1160–1165

Bordron A, Dueymes M, Levy Y, Jamin C, Leroy JP, Piette JC, Shoenfeld Y, Youinou PY (1998) The binding of some human antiendothelial cell antibodies induces endothelial cell apoptosis. J Clin Invest 101:2029–2035

Bordron A, Revelen R, D'Arbonneau F, Dueymes M, Renaudineau Y, Jamin C, Youinou P (2001) Functional heterogeneity of anti-endothelial cell antibodies. Clin Exp Immunol 124:492–501

Chen Y, Inobe J, Marks R, Gonnella P, Kuchroo VK, Weiner HL (1995) Peripheral deletion of antigen-reactive T cells in oral tolerance. Nature 376:177–180

Chen Y, Kuchroo VK, Inobe J, Hafler DA, Weiner HL (1994) Regulatory T cell clones induced by oral tolerance: suppression of autoimmune encephalomyelitis. Science 265:1237–1240

Faria AM, Weiner HL (1999) Oral tolerance: mechanisms and therapeutic applications. Adv Immunol 73:153–264

George J, Meroni PL, Gilburd B, Raschi E, Harats D, Shoenfeld Y (2000) Anti-endothelial cell antibodies in patients with coronary atherosclerosis. Immunol Lett 73:23–27

Groux H, O'Garra A, Bigler M, Rouleau M, Antonenko S, de Vries JE, Roncarolo MG (1997) A CD4+ T-cell subset inhibits antigen-specific T-cell responses and prevents colitis. Nature 389:737–742

Hallenbeck JM, Dutka AJ, Kochanek PM, Sirén A-L, Pezeshkpour GH, Feuerstein G (1988) Stroke risk factors prepare rat brainstem tissues for modified local Shwartzman reaction. Stroke 19:863–869

Hughes CC, Savage CO, Pober JS (1990) The endothelial cell as a regulator of T-cell function. Immunol Rev 117:85–102

Labow MA, Norton CR, Rumberger JM, Lombard-Gillooly KM, Shuster DJ, Hubbard J, Bertko R, Knaack PA, Terry RW, Harbison ML, et al (1994) Characterization of E-selectin-deficient mice: demonstration of overlapping function of the endothelial selectins. Immunity 1:709–720

Libby P, Sukhova G, Lee RT, Galis ZS (1995) Cytokines regulate vascular functions related to stability of the atherosclerotic plaque. J Cardiovasc Pharmacol 25 Suppl 2:S9–12

Liuzzo G, Kopecky SL, Frye RL, O'Fallon WM, Maseri A, Goronzy JJ, Weyand CM (1999) Perturbation of the T-cell repertoire in patients with unstable angina. Circulation 100:2135–2139

McCarron RM, Wang L, Cowan EP, Spatz M (1991) Class II MHC antigen expression by cultured human cerebral vascular endothelial cells. Brain Res 566:325–328

Metzler B, Wraith DC (1996) Mucosal tolerance in a murine model of experimental autoimmune encephalomyelitis. Ann N Y Acad Sci 778:228–242

Miller A, Lider O, Roberts AB, Sporn MB, Weiner HL (1992) Suppressor T cells generated by oral tolerization to myelin basic protein suppress both in vitro and in vivo immune responses by the release of transforming growth factor beta after antigen-specific triggering. Proc Natl Acad Sci U S A 89:421–425

Montgomery KF, Osborn L, Hession C, Tizard R, Goff D, Vassallo C, Tarr PI, Bomsztyk K, Lobb R, Harlan JM, et al (1991) Activation of endothelial-leukocyte adhesion molecule 1 (ELAM-1) gene transcription. Proc Natl Acad Sci U S A 88:6523–6527

Okada Y, Copeland BR, Mori E, Tung M-M, Thomas WS, del Zoppo GJ (1994) P-selectin and intercellular adhesion molecule-1 expression after focal brain ischemia and reperfusion. Stroke 25:202–211

Osborne KA, Shigeno T, Balarsky AM, Ford I, McCulloch J, Teasdale GM, Graham DI (1987) Quantitative assessment of early brain damage in a rat model of focal cerebral ischaemia. J Neurol Neurosurg Psychiat 50:402–410

Pober JS, Cotran RS (1990) Cytokines and endothelial cell biology. Physiol Rev 70:427–451

Prud'homme GJ, Piccirillo CA (2000) The inhibitory effects of transforming growth factor-beta-1 (TGF-beta1) in autoimmune diseases. J Autoimmun 14:23–42

Rosenberg RD, Aird WC (1999) Vascular-bed-specific hemostasis and hypercoagulable states. N Engl J Med 340:1555–1564

Ruetzler CA, Furuya K, Takeda H, Hallenbeck JM (2001) Brain vessels normally undergo cyclic activation and inactivation: evidence from tumor necrosis factor-alpha, heme oxygenase-1, and manganese superoxide dismutase immunostaining of vessels and perivascular brain cells. J Cereb Blood Flow Metab 21:244–252

Salmi M, Granfors K, Leirisalo-Repo M, Hamalainen M, MacDermott R, Leino R, Havia T, Jalkanen S (1992) Selective endothelial binding of interleukin-2-dependent human T-cell lines derived from different tissues. Proc Natl Acad Sci U S A 89:11436–11440

Siren AL, McCarron R, Wang L, Garcia-Pinto P, Ruetzler C, Martin D, Hallenbeck JM (2001) Proinflammatory cytokine expression contributes to brain injury provoked by chronic monocyte activation. Mol Med 7:219–229

von Andrian UH, Mackay CR (2000) T-cell function and migration. Two sides of the same coin. N Engl J Med 343:1020–1034

von Asmuth EJ, Smeets EF, Ginsel LA, Onderwater JJ, Leeuwenberg JF, Buurman WA (1992) Evidence for endocytosis of E-selectin in human endothelial cells. Eur J Immunol 22:2519–2526

Weiner HL (1997) Oral tolerance: immune mechanisms and treatment of autoimmune diseases. Immunol Today 18:335–343

Weyand CM, Goronzy JJ, Liuzzo G, Kopecky SL, Holmes DR, Jr., Frye RL (2001) T-cell immunity in acute coronary syndromes. Mayo Clin Proc 76:1011–1020

Yamori Y, Horie R, Akiguchi I, Kihara M, Nara Y, Lovenberg W (1982) Symptomatological classification in the development of stroke in stroke-prone spontaneously hypertensive rats. Jpn Circ J 46:274–283

Zoldhelyi P, Beck PJ, Bjercke RJ, Ober JC, Hu X, McNatt JM, Akhtar S, Ahmed M, Clubb FJ, Jr., Chen ZQ, Dixon RA, Yeh ET, Willerson JT (2000) Inhibition of coronary thrombosis and local inflammation by a noncarbohydrate selectin inhibitor. Am J Physiol Heart Circ Physiol 279:H3065–3075

8 Protective Autoimmunity and Prospects for Therapeutic Vaccination Against Self-Perpetuating Neurodegeneration

M. Schwartz

8.1 Is Inflammation Good or Bad for Central Nervous System Repair?

Inflammation, although generally accepted as the body's defense mechanism, has received a bad reputation in regard to the central nervous system (CNS). It should be stressed, however, that inflammation is not a single process, but involves cascades of processes mediated by numerous compounds and factors (Hauben et al. 2002; Hauben and Schwartz 2003; Schwartz and Hauben 2003). The function of inflammation in acute or chronic insults to the CNS has long been a matter of debate. Concepts such as the immune-privileged status of the CNS, as well as observations such as the presence of immune cells in the diseased CNS, have helped to foster the belief that immune activity in the CNS is detrimental (Lotan and Schwartz 1994; Hauben and Schwartz 2003). Many authors, for example, consider inflammation to be an important mediator of secondary damage (Constantini and Young 1994; Dusart and Schwab 1994; Carlson et al. 1998; Fitch et al. 1999; Popovich et al. 1999; Mautes et al. 2000; Ghirnikar et al. 2001). On the other hand, studies have shown that inflammation, by promoting clearance of cell debris and secretion of neurotrophic factors and cytokines, may beneficially affect the traumatized spinal cord. Macrophages and microglia promote axonal regeneration (David et al. 1990; Perry and Brown 1992; Rapalino et al. 1998; Fitch et al. 1999; Ousman and David 2001), and T cells mediate processes of maintenance and repair, thus promoting functional recovery from CNS trauma (Moalem et al. 1999b; Hauben et al. 2000a,b; Hausler et al. 2002; Elward and Gasque 2003; Hofstetter et al. 2003; Olsson et al. 2003).

As more pieces are added to the puzzle it becomes increasingly evident that to describe inflammation as a unified event that is "good" or "bad" for the injured nerve is an oversimplification, because it presupposes a single (and deleterious) process rather than a phenomenon with diverse manifestations. In our opinion, inflammation is a series of local immune responses that are recruited to cope with the damage inflicted by an insult, and its ultimate outcome depends upon how it is regulated. Accordingly, the conflicting interpretations of inflammation might reflect the common tendencies to (a) judge parameters (e.g., size of injury, cavitation) other than functional parameters of recovery, (b) evaluate recovery too soon after the injury, and (c) fail to take due account of the species, the strain, and the experimental injury model employed (Kipnis et al. 2001; Hauben et al. 2002; Schori et al. 2002b).

It is also important to recognize that the beneficial effect of immune activity might not come free of charge, i.e., it might come at the expense of some neuronal loss or transient manifestation of autoimmune disease symptoms. The net effect of inflammation depends on the balance between cost and benefit, a ratio that should be evaluated only at steady state. Accordingly, at certain stages of the inflammatory cascade macrophage activity might be destructive, albeit transiently. This might also explain the neuronal loss observed after injection of zymosan (nontoxic yeast particles used to activate macrophages and microglia) into the healthy rat CNS (Fitch et al. 1999; Popovich et al. 1999), or injection of encephalitogenic T cells into naive Lewis rats, known to be susceptible to experimental autoimmune encephalomyelitis (EAE). Thus, the injection of cells or agents that promote inflammatory conditions in healthy animals might cause some tissue loss. The same cells and agents, operating in the traumatized CNS, might promote recovery (Hauben et al. 2000b) and reduce cavitation (Butovsky et al. 2001), and although there is a price to pay (in terms of transient EAE), the cost is outweighed by the benefit.

8.2 Glutamate – A Common Player in Neuronal Death

Glutamate is an essential neurotransmitter in the CNS and plays a key role in cognition, learning, and memory (Fonnum 1984). Synaptic activity causes a transient local increase in glutamate concentrations in the synaptic cleft, and transporter-mediated uptake restores glutamate homeostasis (Danbolt 2001).

Although glutamate is essential for life, its increased concentration under CNS stress makes it toxic to the point of self-destruction. Traumatic injury, toxicity of external biochemical agents, oxidative stress, virus-induced degenerative syndromes, and autoimmune disease can all trigger self-destructive processes in which glutamate is a leading player (Choi 1988). Moreover, glutamate toxicity can lead to oxidative stress via glutamate receptors (McCord 1985; Dumuis et al. 1988; Dawson et al. 1992; Mattammal et al. 1995; Herrera et al. 2001), cystine transporters (Bannai and Kitamura 1980), or lipid peroxidation (Herrera et al. 2001).

Until quite recently, most studies of glutamate clearance or of protection from glutamate toxicity did not assign a role to mechanisms outside the CNS. Any immune involvement either local or systemic, was assumed to be detrimental. Macrophages and microglia were shown to be involved in brain pathology by releasing glutamate

(Piani and Fontana 1994). Interestingly, however, both cell types in-vitro were also shown to express glutamate transporters and take up glutamate (Rimaniol et al. 2000; Nakajima et al. 2001). The associa-tion between ongoing degeneration and the presence of activated mi-croglia/macrophages was usually interpreted as part of the posttrau-matic pathology (Carlson et al. 1999; Appel and Simpson 2001; McGreal et al. 2002; Minagar et al. 2002; Wu du et al. 2002). Accu-mulated findings suggest, however, that this may not necessarily be the case (Kerschensteiner et al. 1999; Moalem et al. 1999b; Hammar-berg et al. 2000; Hohlfeld et al. 2000; Serpe et al. 2000). It is possible that in cases of acute injury or chronic damage to the CNS, the initial activation of microglia, though in principle beneficial, is insufficient to prevent degeneration. Ongoing degeneration in an environment of ac-tivated microglia might thus give the erroneous impression that these cells participate in the etiology rather than the repair. It is also possi-ble that microglia – which like all immune cells can acquire multiple phenotypes (including detrimental ones) – might be recruited within a context which does not allow the optimal phenotype to be acquired. In such a case they might be non-effective or even detrimental. Glutamate is but one example of many self-compounds which, under pathological conditions, are destructive or even infective.

8.3 Protective Autoimmunity – A Physiological Response to CNS Insult

Early studies in rats, using a partial crush injury of the optic nerve or severe spinal cord contusion as a model, showed that systemic in-jection of T cells specific to myelin-associated peptides reduces the postinjury loss of neurons and fibers (Fig. 1). Thus, significantly more retinal ganglion cells (RGCs) survive axonal injury in rats treated with myelin-specific T cells than in rats treated with T cells specific to an irrelevant antigen such as ovalbumin (OVA) or not treated at all (Moalem et al. 1999b). Similar findings were obtained for recovery of motor activity after spinal cord contusion (Moalem et al. 1999b; Hauben et al. 2000a,b). It was further shown that the beneficial effect of the autoimmune T cells on neural tissue is ac-companied by better preservation of the tissue and less cavity forma-tion (Hauben et al. 2000b, 2001, 2003; Butovsky et al. 2001).

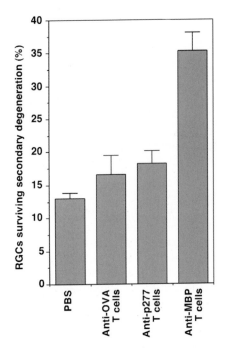

Fig. 1. T cells specific to myelin basic protein (*MBP*), but not to the irrelevant antigens ovalbumin (*OVA*) or p277 of hsp60, protect neurons from secondary degeneration. Immediately after partial crush injury to the optic nerve, rats were injected with anti-MBP, anti-OVA, or anti-p277 T cells, or with PBS nontreated. The neurotracer dye 4-Di-10-Asp was applied to the nerve distally to the site of the lesion, either immediately after injury (for assessment of primary damage) or 2 weeks later (for assessment of secondary degeneration). Five days after dye application, the retinas were excised and flat-mounted. Labeled RGCs from 3–5 randomly selected fields in each retina (all located at approx. the same distance from the optic disk) were counted under a fluorescence microscope. The number of surviving RGCs in each treatment group was expressed as a percentage of the total number of RGCs that escaped the primary injury The neuroprotective effect of the anti-MBP T cells compared to that of PBS was significant ($P < 0.001$, one-way ANOVA). Anti-OVA T cells and anti-p277 T cells did not differ significantly from PBS in their protective effects on neurons that had escaped the primary injury ($P > 0.05$, one-way ANOVA). The results are a summary of five experiments. Each group contained 5 to 10 rats. (After Moalem et al. 1999b)

8.4 Antigenic Specificity of Protective Autoimmunity

In studies aimed at determining whether the observed beneficial effect is a physiological phenomenon, our group concluded that injury to CNS myelinated axons spontaneously evokes a systemic T cell-mediated response that reduces the spread of damage. In the absence of T cells, recovery is worse (Kipnis et al. 2001; Yoles et al. 2001). Protection occurred even in cases where the autoimmune T cells caused a transient autoimmune disease (Moalem et al. 1999b; Hauben et al. 2000a). Interestingly, some strains were less able than others to spontaneously manifest a protective response, a phenomenon that we attribute not to the presence of a destructive mechanism but to the relative impotence of the protective mechanism (Kipnis et al. 2001). Recently we demonstrated that neonatally induced tolerance to myelin antigens reduces the adult rat's ability to withstand axonal injury, indicating that the T cell-dependent protection which is spontaneously evoked in response to an injury to myelinated axons is myelin-specific (Kipnis et al. 2002a,b). Paradoxically, after a CNS insult, strains that are inherently more susceptible to autoimmune disease were more limited in their ability to spontaneously manifest the T cell-mediated neuroprotection. As discussed below, this limitation in part reflects the efficacy of regulation of the autoimmune response (Kipnis et al. 2000).

We attempted to determine whether a T cell-mediated response is also spontaneously manifested after an insult caused directly by glutamate exposure, and if so, whether it can effectively protect the affected site against the consequences of the insult (Schori et al. 2001b). Intraocular injection of glutamate into the vitreous of mice resulted in significantly higher glutamate toxicity if the mice were deprived of T cells (Schori et al. 2001b) (Fig. 2). As in the case of axonal injury, strains differed in their ability to withstand the consequences of the insult (Kipnis et al. 2001; Schori et al. 2001b). Thus, T cell deprivation hardly affected the postinjury neuronal loss in strains with low constitutional resistance to glutamate toxicity, but caused substantial loss in more resistant strains. These studies (Kipnis et al. 2001; Schori et al. 2001b) provided the first demonstration that local coping mechanisms against glutamate insult are assisted by a systemic immune response. The unexpected observation that

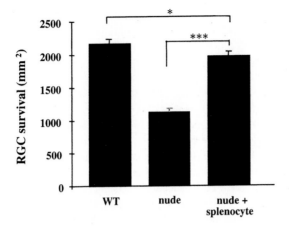

Fig. 2. Splenocytes from wild-type mice can compensate for glutamate-induced neuronal loss in T cell-deficient mice. Wild-type and nude BALB/c mice were injected intravitreally with 200 nmol glutamate. The nude mice also received intravenous injections of 3×10^7–4×10^7 splenocytes from naive BALB/c wild-type mice. After 7 days, RGCs were counted as described. RGC loss in glutamate-injected nude mice that also received splenocytes ($n=10$) was significantly smaller than in glutamate-injected nude mice not supplied with splenocytes ($n=6$; $P<0.0019$, Student's t test). It should be noted, however, that reconstitution with splenocytes under our experimental conditions was not complete, as the numbers of surviving RGCs in the splenocyte-injected nude mice ($n=6$) were still smaller than in the wild-type mice ($n=13$; $P<0.04$, Student's t-test). (After Schori et al. 2001a)

the body's immune response can assist the overburdened local coping mechanisms of the CNS led us to extend the traditional view of immune system function as protection against foreign invaders (such as microorganisms) to include protection against the toxicity of self-derived compounds, i.e., against the enemy within (Schori et al. 2001b, 2002; Schwartz and Kipnis 2001, 2002b; Nevo et al. 2003). The strain-related dependence of glutamate-induced toxicity was found to apply not only to the extent of toxicity but also to the mechanism underlying the toxicity, as shown by the response to treatment with receptor antagonists (Schori et al. 2002).

The discovery that glutamate toxicity is dependent on T cells specific to self-antigens prompted our group to search for a way to boost this response as a means of reducing glutamate toxicity. On the basis of our earlier experience with axonal injury of the optic nerve (Fisher et al. 2001), the antigens we chose were proteins and peptides associated with myelin. The results indicated, however, that for stress sites containing no myelin, such as the eye (Schori et al. 2001 b; Mizrahi et al. 2002), this was not the right choice. In retrospect we realized that these antigens could not be effective, because the T cells function only after homing to the site of damage and becoming activated when they encounter their relevant antigens there. It was therefore not surprising to discover that the T cell-dependent resistance to intraocular glutamate toxicity could be boosted by vaccination with antigens that are abundantly expressed in the eye (Mizrahi et al. 2002) (Fig. 3). An example of such an antigen is a pathogenic peptide derived from the interphotoreceptor retinoid binding protein (IRBP) (Avichezer et al. 2000; Adamus and Chan 2002). This peptide is recognized as a contributory factor in the etiology of experimental autoimmune uveitis (EAU), an ocular autoimmune disease. It therefore seems that a peptide which boosts beneficial autoimmunity at the site of stress (Mizrahi et al. 2002) is also potentially capable of inducing an autoimmune disease at that site (Fauser et al. 2001). We found that protection from glutamate toxicity in the rat eye is not restricted to IRBP, as two other uveitogenic peptides, both derived from the retinal protein S-antigen, exerted similar protective effects. Moreover, vaccination with IRBP-peptide analogs designed to evoke an immune response without causing disease also increased RGC survival, indicating that nonpathogenic antigens derived from a pathogenic peptide can be used to protect RGCs from insult-induced death without risk of inducing an autoimmune disease (Fisher et al. 2001; Hauben et al. 2001; Mizrahi et al. 2002).

The same principle was found to apply in the case of damage to myelinated axons, where protective myelin antigens such as myelin basic protein (MBP) or myelin oligodendrocyte glycoprotein (MOG) were also associated with myelin-related autoimmune disease (Moalem et al. 1999b; Fisher et al. 2001). In both cases, nonpathogenic cryptic peptides derived from the same immunodominant proteins induced protective autoimmunity without inducing the disease (Moalem et al. 1999b; Fisher et al. 2001; Mizrahi et al. 2002). These and

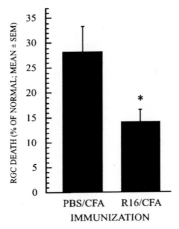

Fig. 3. Immunization with R16 protects RGCs from glutamate toxicity in Lewis rats. RGCs of adult Lewis rats were exposed directly to glutamate toxicity by intravitreal injection of L-glutamate (400 nmol). Immediately thereafter the rats were immunized with 30 μg of R16 emulsified in complete Freund's adjuvant (*CFA*; 0.5 mg/ml). Control rats were injected with PBS in CFA. Two weeks later the optic nerves were exposed for the second time, and the fluorescent dye 4-Di-10-Asp was applied distally to the injury site. Five days after dye application the retinas were detached from the eyes and prepared as flattened whole mounts. Labeled RGCs from four randomly selected fields of identical size in each retina (all located at approximately the same distance from the optic disk) were counted under a fluorescence microscope, and the RGC loss was calculated and expressed as a percentage of (mean±SEM). RGC loss was significantly smaller in the R16-immunized rats than in their matched PBS-injected controls (14±2% and 28±4%, respectively, $P<0.04$; two-tailed Student's t-test). Each group contained five or six rats. (After Mizrahi et al. 2002)

other observations support our proposed concept of protective autoimmunity (Moalem et al. 1999b) as the body's rigorously controlled mechanism of repair.

Neonatal immunization with a homogenate of retinal proteins apparently deprived mice [endowed with the spontaneous ability to harness protective autoimmunity (e.g. BALB/c)] of the ability to manifest an immune response to the abundant eye proteins as adults (Avidan et al., unpublished observations). These findings further substantiate our contention that the physiological protective response is directed against abundant proteins residing at the site of stress (Kipnis et al. 2002 b).

In our view, the threatened tissue endangers some cells for the purpose of saving others. We suggest that the relevant antigen evokes an autoimmune response which, in the event of malfunction, induces disease, but not necessarily in the directly threatened cells such as the RGCs in uveitis or myelinated CNS axons in EAE. Nevertheless, in the absence of appropriate regulation, the autoimmune response might eventually lead to neuronal loss as well. Accumulating information indicates that autoimmune diseases in humans are often accompanied by neuronal loss and an increase in glutamate (Bjartmar et al. 2001; Bjartmar and Trapp 2001; De Stefano et al. 2001; Steinman 2001; Schwartz and Kipnis 2002 a).

8.5 Regulation of Protective Autoimmunity and the Mechanism Underlying It

Our data show that proinflammatory autoimmune T helper cells (Th1) mediate protection against the consequences of CNS insults (Kipnis et al. 2002 a). Thus, paradoxically, the T cells that protect against CNS insults have the same phenotype as those implicated in the pathogenesis of autoimmune disease. The difference in their effects apparently lies in their regulation (Kipnis et al. 2002 b), as well as in the specificity of the response to epitopes within the same protein. Thus, whereas Th1 cells specific to a cryptic epitope (Moalem et al. 1999 b; Fisher et al. 2001) or a modified pathogenic epitope (Hauben et al. 2001) are protective, Th1 cells specific to a pathogenic epitope within the same protein may be both protective and destructive (Moalem et al. 1999 b; Fisher et al. 2001).

Prior to our studies, the prevailing notion was that the naturally occurring regulatory T cells known as $CD4^+CD25^+$ cells are part of the mechanism through which the body maintains non-responsiveness to self and thus prevents development of autoimmune disease. In our view, the function of these regulatory T cells is to endow an individual with the ability tolerate response to self-antigens needed for neuronal protection, without developing autoimmune diseases

(Schwartz and Kipnis 2002b). We further postulated that the presence of these regulatory T cells allows differential activation of some but not all of the autoimmune effector T cells (Kipnis et al. 2002b) (Fig. 4). When protective autoimmunity functions properly (as in strains resistant to injurious conditions), the regulatory T cells apparently allow early selective activation of only those autoimmune T cells that do not carry the risk of autoimmune disease (Schwartz and Kipnis 2002b). Rats or mice of strains that are resistant to autoimmune disease development, and when deprived of $CD4^+CD25^+$ regulatory T cells, are better able to withstand the consequences of optic nerve injury than normal EAE-resistant strains. The increase in ability to withstand an insult (Schwartz and Kipnis 2002b) after removal of $CD4^+CD25^+$ cells is inevitably accompanied by an increased likelihood of autoimmune disease development (Shevach 2002). Recent studies suggest that when mice that are relatively resistant to glutamate toxicity receive $CD4^+CD25^+$ cells isolated from wild-type matched controls, they lose the advantage of resistance to the effects of both mechanical injury (Kipnis et al. 2002b) and glutamate toxicity (Kipnis et al., unpublished observations).

Interestingly, the efficacy of the autoimmune response in helping the body to resist cancer development has also been linked to $CD4^+CD25^+$ regulatory T cells. We postulate that the regulatory T cells are the cells that determine the risk/benefit ratio, i.e., that they allow a protective anti-self response to be manifested without running the risk of autoimmune disease induction. When autoimmune effector cells are needed for protective activity, their switch-on and switch-off is controlled by the regulatory activity of the $CD4^+CD25^+$ T cells. We recently discovered that a stress-related compound produced by the CNS can block the suppressive activity of the regulatory T cells, a prerequisite for recruiting an anti-self response (Kipnis et al., unpublished observations). This compound is a key player in the most upstream event in the cascade of reactions needed to harness a protective response.

In further studies of how the autoimmune T cells display their protective effect, we observed that the microglia appear to act as an intermediary between the systemic immune response and local toxicity. This observation led us to view the microglia as stand-by cells, potentially capable of displaying both immune activity and neural activity as required. This further substantiates our assumption that anti-self T cells act as helper T cells (Th1) when called upon to do so. We examined whether microglia, under stressful conditions, can display dual activity, serving as both antigen-presenting cells (in the context of the immune dialog), and as buffer cells (a nerve-related activity). Given our earlier results showing that after CNS insult the injury site is depleted of astrocytes (the usual buffering cells) (Blaugrund et al. 1993) and repopulated by macrophages/microglia

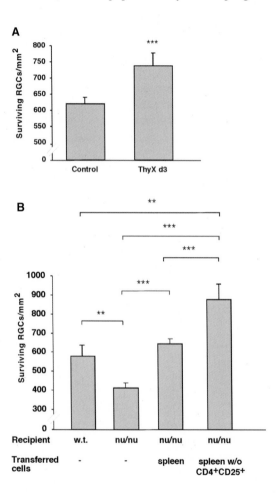

(Hirschberg et al. 1994; Moalem et al. 1999a; Butovsky et al. 2001), this seemed feasible. Moreover, our in vitro studies demonstrated that, like antigen-presenting cells, microglia exposed to activated T cells show an increase in class II major histocompatibility complex proteins and the costimulatory molecule B.7.2, as well as an increased capacity for glutamate uptake (Shaked et al., unpublished observations). The effect of T cells on buffering capacity could be reproduced by adding IFN-γ to the cultured microglia (Shaked et al., unpublished observations). Gene array analysis demonstrated that activation of microglia by activated T cells led to upregulation of a cluster of genes associated with an increased ability to resist oxidative stress (Shaked et al., unpublished observations).

8.6 A Therapeutic Vaccine for Neurodegenerative Diseases

In designing and developing therapy for glutamate-associated neurodegenerative diseases, our approach is based on the concept that a well-controlled autoimmune response, if directed against antigens residing at the site of stress and expressed at the right time, can

Fig. 4A,B. Deprivation of naturally occurring regulatory CD4$^+$CD25$^+$ T cells in BALB/c mice improves neuronal survival after optic nerve crush injury. **A** BALB/c mice were thymectomized 3 days after birth to deprive them of regulatory T cells, and were subjected as adults to severe unilateral crush injury inflicted on the intraorbital portion of the optic nerve. Surviving neurons were labeled by the application, 3 days prior to injury, of the neurotracer dye FluoroGold. Significantly more neurons survived in the thymectomized mice than in age-matched nonthymectomized controls ($n=7$–8 in each group; $P<0.001$; Student's t-test). **B** Neuronal survival after optic nerve crush injury in BALB/c nu/nu mice (devoid of T cells) was worse than in wild-type mice of matched background. Endogenous neuroprotection in the nude mice was restored by injection of 5×10^7 splenocytes. Injection of splenocytes deprived of regulatory CD4$^+$CD25$^+$ T cells increased neuronal survival in these mice beyond that seen in the wild type ($n=5$–6 in each group; P values between different groups, obtained by two-tailed Student's t test, are indicated by *asterisks above the graph bars*; * $P<0.05$; ** $P<0.01$; *** $P<0.001$). (After Schwartz and Kipnis 2002b)

benefit stressed tissue without inducing an autoimmune disease (Schwartz and Kipnis 2001, 2002 a, c; Kipnis and Schwartz 2002).

Our experiments in rats and mice showed that vaccination with the synthetic polymer Cop-1 (Arnon et al. 1996; Aharoni et al. 1997; Sela and Teitelbaum 2001) apparently results in low-affinity activation of a wide range of self-reactive T cells (Hafler 2002; Kipnis and Schwartz 2002), and can boost the T cell effect, achieving autoimmunity reminiscent of that conferred by cryptic epitopes. Thus, after optic nerve injury or exposure to glutamate toxicity, immunization of rats with Cop-1 protected their RGCs from insult-induced death. This finding suggested that Cop-1 circumvents at least part of the tissue-specificity barrier, and encouraged us to examine whether this copolymer is effective in chronic neurodegenerative conditions. One such disease is glaucoma, a chronic neurodegenerative disease of the optic nerve (Bakalash et al. 2003; Schori et al. 2001 b).

Because the proposed therapy is based on a concept and not on indications, the same therapeutic approach can be applied in a wide range of indications. As mentioned earlier, the vaccination is directed not against the threatening compounds but against antigens residing at the site of stress. Since Cop-1 circumvents the site-specificity barrier due to its ability to weakly cross-react with a wide range of self-compounds, its use has been extended to numerous models, including head trauma (Kipnis et al. 2003), amyotrophic lateral sclerosis (ALS) and acute motor dysfunction (Angelov et al. 2003), and Huntington's disease (Schori et al., unpublished observations) (Fig. 5).

In the case of ALS, for example, it was shown that at least part of the motor neuron loss is attributable to a deficiency in glutamate transporters (Maragakis and Rothstein 2001; Howland et al. 2002). This finding prompted us to examine whether Cop-1 can protect motor neurons in a mouse model of chronic ALS (Angelov et al. 2003). The results suggest that Cop-1 vaccination, in a protocol different from that currently approved and used for patients with multiple sclerosis (MS), can slow down ALS progression, thereby increasing the lifespan of transgenic mice expressing the human SOD1 defective gene. These results substantiate our hypothesis that autoimmune disease and neurodegenerative disorders are two extreme manifestations of a common risk factor, and accordingly that therapy should

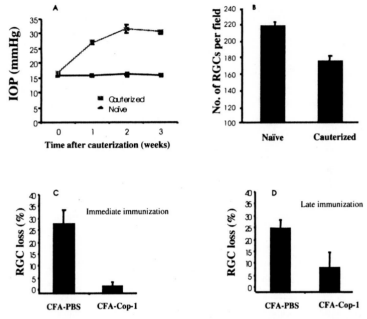

Fig. 5 A–D. Effects of chronically increased intraocular pressure (*IOP*) and Cop-1 immunization on RGC survival in Lewis rats. **A** Laser cauterization causing occlusion of the episcleral and limbal veins results in an increase in IOP and subsequent death of RGCs. Three weeks after laser treatment, the mean IOP was 30.4 ± 0.42 mmHg (mean$\pm$SEM, $n=5$) in rats subjected to venous occlusion and 15.8 ± 0.2 mmHg ($n=7$) in naïve rats. **B** Three weeks after venous occlusion, surviving RGCs were counted in the laser-treated rats and in naïve rats (bars represent mean$\pm$SEM). **C** Rats were immunized with Cop-1 ($n=15$) or injected with PBS ($n=13$) in CFA immediately after laser cauterization. Bars represent RGC loss, calculated as a percentage of the number of RGCs in naïve rats (mean$\pm$SEM). The difference between the numbers of RGCs in the two groups was significant ($P<0.002$, two-tailed Student's t-test). **D** Ten days after venous occlusion the rats were immunized with either Cop-1 ($n=5$) or PBS ($n=4$). Bars represent RGC loss, calculated as a percentage of the number of RGCs (mean$\pm$SEM) in naïve animals. A tendency toward a neuroprotective effect was observed even after delayed immunization with Cop-1; the difference between the numbers of RGCs in the two groups in this case was significant only when assessed by a one-tailed t-test ($P=0.04$). (After Schori et al. 2001 b)

be based not on immune suppression but on immune modulation (Kipnis and Schwartz 2002).

8.7 Concluding Remarks

Our findings show for the first time that CNS homeostasis is controlled not only locally, but also systemically by the adaptive arm of the immune response directed against antigens residing at the site of glutamate stress. They provide the first direct evidence that stress-induced immune responses mediate an ongoing dialog between T cells and CNS tissue. As glutamate is a key player in brain activity, and lack of its proper regulation is a key factor in cognitive, neural, psychogenic, and neurodegenerative disorders, the novel concept of immune system participation in glutamate regulation might represent a landmark in our understanding of how the body controls the brain and in the development of therapies for not only an excess but also a deficiency of glutamate.

Acknowledgments. We thank S. Smith for editing the manuscript. M.S. holds the Maurice and Ilse Katz Professorial Chair in Neuroimmunology. The work was supported by Proneuron Ltd., Industrial Park, Ness-Ziona, Israel and in part by grants from The Glaucoma Research Foundation and The Alan Brown Foundation for Spinal Cord Injury awarded to M.S.

References

Adamus G, Chan CC (2002) Experimental autoimmune uveitides: multiple antigens, diverse diseases. Int Rev Immunol 21:209–229
Aharoni R, Teitelbaum D, Sela M, Arnon R (1997) Copolymer 1 induces T cells of the T helper type 2 that crossreact with myelin basic protein and suppress experimental autoimmune encephalomyelitis. Proc Natl Acad Sci USA 94:10821–10826
Angelov DN, Waibel S, Guntinas-Lichius O, Lenzen M, Neiss WF, Tomov TL, Yoles E, Kipnis J, Schori H, Reuter A, Ludolph A, Schwartz M (2003) Therapeutic vaccine for acute and chronic motor neuron diseases: Implications for ALS. Proc Natl Acad Sci USA 100:4790–4795

Appel SH, Simpson EP (2001) Activated microglia: the silent executioner in neurodegenerative disease? Curr Neurol Neurosci Rep 1:303–305

Arnon R, Sela M, Teitelbaum D (1996) New insights into the mechanism of action of copolymer 1 in experimental allergic encephalomyelitis and multiple sclerosis. J Neurol 243:S8–13

Avichezer D, Chan CC, Silver PB, Wiggert B, Caspi RR (2000) Residues 1–20 of IRBP and whole IRBP elicit different uveitogenic and immunological responses in interferon gamma deficient mice. Exp Eye Res 71:111–118

Bakalash S, Kessler A, Mizrahi T, Nussenblatt R, Schwartz M (2003) Antigenic specificity of immunoprotective therapeutic vaccination for glaucoma. Invest Ophthalmol Vis Sci 44:3374–3381

Bannai S, Kitamura E (1980) Transport interaction of L-cystine and L-glutamate in human diploid fibroblasts in culture. J Biol Chem 255:2372–2376

Bjartmar C, Trapp BD (2001) Axonal and neuronal degeneration in multiple sclerosis: mechanisms and functional consequences. Curr Opin Neurol 14:271–278

Bjartmar C, Kinkel RP, Kidd G, Rudick RA, Trapp BD (2001) Axonal loss in normal-appearing white matter in a patient with acute MS. Neurology 57:1248–1252

Blaugrund E, Lavie V, Cohen I, Solomon A, Schreyer DJ, Schwartz M (1993) Axonal regeneration is associated with glial migration: comparison between the injured optic nerves of fish and rats. J Comp Neurol 330:105–112

Butovsky O, Hauben E, Schwartz M (2001) Morphological aspects of spinal cord autoimmune neuroprotection: colocalization of T cells with B7–2 (CD86) and prevention of cyst formation. Faseb J 15:1065–1067

Carlson NG, Wieggel WA, Chen J, Bacchi A, Rogers SW, Gahring LC (1999) Inflammatory cytokines IL-1 alpha, IL-1 beta, IL-6, and TNF-alpha impart neuroprotection to an excitotoxin through distinct pathways. J Immunol 163:3963–3968

Carlson SL, Parrish ME, Springer JE, Doty K, Dossett L (1998) Acute inflammatory response in spinal cord following impact injury. Exp Neurol 151:77–88

Choi DW (1988) Glutamate neurotoxicity and diseases of the nervous system. Neuron 1:623–634

Constantini S, Young W (1994) The effects of methylprednisolone and the ganglioside GM1 on acute spinal cord injury in rats. J Neurosurg 80:97–111

Danbolt NC (2001) Glutamate uptake. Prog Neurobiol 65:1–105

David S, Bouchard C, Tsatas O, Giftochristos N (1990) Macrophages can modify the nonpermissive nature of the adult mammalian central nervous system. Neuron 5:463–469

Dawson TM, Dawson VL, Snyder SH (1992) A novel neuronal messenger molecule in brain: the free radical, nitric oxide. Ann Neurol 32:297–311; Comment in: Ann Neurol 1993; 1933(1994):1422

De Stefano N, Narayanan S, Francis GS, Arnaoutelis R, Tartaglia MC, Antel JP, Matthews PM, Arnold DL (2001) Evidence of axonal damage in the early stages of multiple sclerosis and its relevance to disability. Arch Neurol 58:65–70

Dumuis A, Sebben M, Haynes L, Pin JP, Bockaert J (1988) NMDA receptors activate the arachidonic acid cascade system in striatal neurons. Nature 336:68–70

Dusart I, Schwab ME (1994) Secondary cell death and the inflammatory reaction after dorsal hemisection of the rat spinal cord. Eur J Neurosci 6:712–724

Fauser S, Nguyen TD, Bekure K, Schluesener HJ, Meyermann R (2001) Differential activation of microglial cells in local and remote areas of IRBP1169–1191-induced rat uveitis. Acta Neuropathol (Berl) 101:565–571

Fisher J, Levkovitch-Verbin H, Schori H, Yoles E, Butovsky O, Kaye JF, Ben-Nun A, Schwartz M (2001) Vaccination for neuroprotection in the mouse optic nerve: implications for optic neuropathies. J Neurosci 21:136–142

Fitch MT, Doller C, Combs CK, Landreth GE, Silver J (1999) Cellular and molecular mechanisms of glial scarring and progressive cavitation: in vivo and in vitro analysis of inflammation-induced secondary injury after CNS trauma. J Neurosci 19:8182–8198

Fonnum F (1984) Glutamate: a neurotransmitter in mammalian brain. J Neurochem 42:1–11

Ghirnikar RS, Lee YL, Eng LF (2001) Chemokine antagonist infusion promotes axonal sparing after spinal cord contusion injury in rat. J Neurosci Res 64:582–589

Hafler DA (2002) Degeneracy, as opposed to specificity, in immunotherapy. J Clin Invest 109:581–584

Hammarberg H, Lidman O, Lundberg C, Eltayeb SY, Gielen AW, Muhallab S, Svenningsson A, Linda H, van der Meide PH, Cullheim S, Olsson T, Piehl F (2000) Neuroprotection by encephalomyelitis: rescue of mechanically injured neurons and neurotrophin production by CNS-infiltrating T and natural killer cells. J Neurosci 20:5283–5291

Hauben E, Nevo U, Yoles E, Moalem G, Agranov E, Mor F, Akselrod S, Neeman M, Cohen IR, Schwartz M (2000a) Autoimmune T cells as potential neuroprotective therapy for spinal cord injury. Lancet 355:286–287

Hauben E, Butovsky O, Nevo U, Yoles E, Moalem G, Agranov E, Mor F, Leibowitz-Amit R, Pevsner E, Akselrod S, Neeman M, Cohen IR, Schwartz M (2000b) Passive or active immunization with myelin basic protein promotes recovery from spinal cord contusion. J Neurosci 20: 6421–6430

Hauben E, Agranov E, Gothilf A, Nevo U, Cohen A, Smirnov I, Steinman L, Schwartz M (2001) Posttraumatic therapeutic vaccination with modified myelin self-antigen prevents complete paralysis while avoiding autoimmune disease. J Clin Invest 108:591–599

Hauben E, Mizrahi T, Agranov E, Schwartz M (2002) Sexual dimorphism in the spontaneous recovery from spinal cord injury: a gender gap in beneficial autoimmunity? Eur J Neurosci 16:1731–1740

Hauben E, Schwartz M (2003) Therapeutic vaccination for spinal cord injury: Helping the body to cure itself. Trends Pharmacol Sci 24:7–12

Hauben E, Gothilf A, Cohen A, Butovsky O, Nevo U, Smirnov I, Yoles E, Akselrod S, Schwartz M (2003) Vaccination with dendritic cells pulsed with peptides of myelin basic protein promotes functional recovery from the spinal cord injury. J Neurosci: in press

Herrera F, Sainz RM, Mayo JC, Martin V, Antolin I, Rodriguez C (2001) Glutamate induces oxidative stress not mediated by glutamate receptors or cystine transporters: protective effect of melatonin and other antioxidants. J Pineal Res 31:356–362

Hirschberg DL, Yoles E, Belkin M, Schwartz M (1994) Inflammation after axonal injury has conflicting consequences for recovery of function: rescue of spared axons is impaired but regeneration is supported. J Neuroimmunol 50:9–16

Hohlfeld R, Kerschensteiner M, Stadelmann C, Lassmann H, Wekerle H (2000) The neuroprotective effect of inflammation: implications for the therapy of multiple sclerosis. J Neuroimmunol 107:161–166

Howland DS, Liu J, She Y, Goad B, Maragakis NJ, Kim B, Erickson J, Kulik J, DeVito L, Psaltis G, DeGennaro LJ, Cleveland DW, Rothstein JD (2002) Focal loss of the glutamate transporter EAAT2 in a transgenic rat model of SOD1 mutant-mediated amyotrophic lateral sclerosis (ALS). Proc Natl Acad Sci USA 99:1604–1609

Kerschensteiner M, Gallmeier E, Behrens L, Leal VV, Misgeld T, Klinkert WE, Kolbeck R, Hoppe E, Oropeza-Wekerle RL, Bartke I, Stadelmann C, Lassmann H, Wekerle H, Hohlfeld R (1999) Activated human T cells, B cells, and monocytes produce brain-derived neurotrophic factor in vitro and in inflammatory brain lesions: a neuroprotective role of inflammation? J Exp Med 189:865–870

Kipnis J, Yoles E, Schori H, Hauben E, Shaked I, Schwartz M (2001) Neuronal survival after CNS insult is determined by a genetically encoded autoimmune response. J Neurosci 21:4564–4571

Kipnis J, Schwartz M (2002) Dual action of glatiramer acetate (Cop-1) in the treatment of CNS autoimmune and neurodegenerative disorders. Trends Mol Med 8:319–323

Kipnis J, Mizrahi T, Yoles E, Ben-Nun A, Schwartz M (2002a) Myelin specific Th1 cells are necessary for post-traumatic protective autoimmunity. J Neuroimmunol 130:78–85

Kipnis J, Mizrahi T, Hauben E, Shaked I, Shevach E, Schwartz M (2002b) Neuroprotective autoimmunity: Naturally occurring CD4+CD25+ regulatory T cells suppress the ability to withstand injury to the central nervous system. Proc Natl Acad Sci USA 99:15620–15625

Kipnis J, Yoles E, Porat Z, Cohen A, Mor F, Sela M, Cohen IR, Schwartz M (2000) T cell immunity to copolymer 1 confers neuroprotection on the damaged optic nerve: possible therapy for optic neuropathies. Proc Natl Acad Sci U S A 97:7446–7451

Kipnis J, Nevo U, Panikashvili D, Alexanderovich A, Yoles E, Akselrod S, Shohami E, Schwartz M (2003) Therapeutic Vaccination for Closed Head Injury. J Neurotrauma 20:559–569

Lotan M, Schwartz M (1994) Cross talk between the immune system and the nervous system in response to injury: implications for regeneration. FASEB J 8:1026–1033

Maragakis NJ, Rothstein JD (2001) Glutamate transporters in neurologic disease. Arch Neurol 58:365–370

Mattammal MB, Strong R, Lakshmi VM, Chung HD, Stephenson AH (1995) Prostaglandin H synthetase-mediated metabolism of dopamine: implication for Parkinson's disease. J Neurochem 64:1645–1654

Mautes AE, Weinzierl MR, Donovan F, Noble LJ (2000) Vascular events after spinal cord injury: contribution to secondary pathogenesis. Phys Ther 80:673–687

McCord JM (1985) Oxygen-derived free radicals in postischemic tissue injury. N Engl J Med 312:159–163

McGreal EP, Ikewaki N, Akatsu H, Morgan BP, Gasque P (2002) Human C1qRp is identical with CD93 and the mNI-11 antigen but does not bind C1q. J Immunol 168:5222–5232

Minagar A, Shapshak P, Fujimura R, Ownby R, Heyes M, Eisdorfer C (2002) The role of macrophage/microglia and astrocytes in the pathogenesis of three neurologic disorders: HIV-associated dementia, Alzheimer disease, and multiple sclerosis. J Neurol Sci 202:13–23

Mizrahi T, Hauben E, Schwartz M (2002) The tissue-specific self-pathogen is the protective self-antigen: The case of uveitis. J Immunol 169:5971–5977

Moalem G, Monsonego A, Shani Y, Cohen IR, Schwartz M (1999a) Differential T cell response in central and peripheral nerve injury: connection with immune privilege. Faseb J 13:1207–1217

Moalem G, Leibowitz-Amit R, Yoles E, Mor F, Cohen IR, Schwartz M (1999b) Autoimmune T cells protect neurons from secondary degeneration after central nervous system axotomy. Nat Med 5:49–55

Nakajima K, Tohyama Y, Kohsaka S, Kurihara T (2001) Ability of rat microglia to uptake extracellular glutamate. Neurosci Lett 307:171–174

Nevo U, Hauben E, Yoles E, Agranov E, Akselrod S, Schwartz M, Neeman M (2001) Diffusion anisotropy MRI for quantitative assessment of recovery in injured rat spinal cord. Magn Reson Med 45:1–9

Nevo U, Kipnis J, Golding I, Shaked I, Neumann A, Akselrod S, Schwartz M (2003) Autoimmunity as a special case of immunity: removing threats from within. Trends Mol Med 9:88–93

Ousman SS, David S (2001) MIP-1alpha, MCP-1, GM-CSF, and TNF-alpha control the immune cell response that mediates rapid phagocytosis of myelin from the adult mouse spinal cord. J Neurosci 21:4649–4656

Perry VH, Brown MC (1992) Macrophages and nerve regeneration. Curr Opin Neurobiol 2:679–682

Piani D, Fontana A (1994) Involvement of the cystine transport system xc- in the macrophage-induced glutamate-dependent cytotoxicity to neurons. J Immunol 152:3578–3585

Popovich PG, Guan Z, Wei P, Huitinga I, van Rooijen N, Stokes BT (1999) Depletion of hematogenous macrophages promotes partial hindlimb recovery and neuroanatomical repair after experimental spinal cord injury. Exp Neurol 158:351–365

Rapalino O, Lazarov-Spiegler O, Agranov E, Velan GJ, Yoles E, Fraidakis M, Solomon A, Gepstein R, Katz A, Belkin M, Hadani M, Schwartz M (1998) Implantation of stimulated homologous macrophages results in partial recovery of paraplegic rats. Nat Med 4:814–821

Rimaniol AC, Haik S, Martin M, Le Grand R, Boussin FD, Dereuddre-Bosquet N, Gras G, Dormont D (2000) Na+-dependent high-affinity glutamate transport in macrophages. J Immunol 164:5430–5438

Schori H, Yoles E, Schwartz M (2001a) T-cell-based immunity counteracts the potential toxicity of glutamate in the central nervous system. J Neuroimmunol 119:199–204

Schori H, Kipnis J, Yoles E, WoldeMussie E, Ruiz G, Wheeler LA, Schwartz M (2001b) Vaccination for protection of retinal ganglion cells against death from glutamate cytotoxicity and ocular hypertension: implications for glaucoma. Proc Natl Acad Sci USA 98:3398–3403

Schori H, Lantner F, Shachar I, Schwartz M (2002) Severe immunodeficiency has opposite effects on neuronal survival in glutamate-susceptible and -resistant mice: Adverse effect of B cells. J Immunol 196:2861–2865

Schori H, Yoles E, Wheeler LA, Schwartz M (2002) Immune related mechanisms participating in resistance and susceptibility to glutamate toxicity. Eur J Neurosci 16:557–564

Schwartz M, Kipnis J (2001) Protective autoimmunity: regulation and prospects for vaccination after brain and spinal cord injuries. Trends Mol Med 7:252–258

Schwartz M, Kipnis J (2002) Prospects for therapeutic vaccination with glatiramer acetate for neurodegenerative diseases such as Alzheimer's disease. Drug Dev Res 56:143–149

Schwartz M, Kipnis J (2002a) Multiple sclerosis as a by-product of the failure to sustain protective autoimmunity: A paradigm shift. The Neuroscientist 8:405–413

Schwartz M, Kipnis J (2002b) Autoimmunity on alert: naturally occurring regulatory CD4+CD25+ T cells as part of the evolutionary compromise between a "need" and a "risk". Trends Immunol 23:530–534

Schwartz M, Kipnis J (2003) Harm or heal – divergent effects of autoimmune neuroinflammation? Response from Schwartz and Kipnis. Trends Immunol 24:7–8

Sela M, Teitelbaum D (2001) Glatiramer acetate in the treatment of multiple sclerosis. Expert Opin Pharmacother 2:1149–1165

Serpe CJ, Sanders VM, Jones KJ (2000) Kinetics of facial motoneuron loss following facial nerve transection in severe combined immunodeficient mice [In Process Citation]. J Neurosci Res 62:273–278

Shevach EM (2002) CD4+CD25+ suppressor T cells: more questions than answers. Nat Rev Immunol 2:389–400

Steinman L (2001) Multiple sclerosis: a two-stage disease. Nat Immunol 2:762–764

Wu du C, Tieu K, Cohen O, Choi DK, Vila M, Jackson-Lewis V, Teismann P, Przedborski S (2002) Glial cell response: A pathogenic factor in Parkinson's disease. J Neurovirol 8:551–558

Yoles E, Hauben E, Palgi O, Agranov E, Gothilf A, Cohen A, Kuchroo V, Cohen IR, Weiner H, Schwartz M (2001) Protective autoimmunity is a physiological response to CNS trauma. J Neurosci 21:3740–3748

9 Lessons from Stroke Trials Using Anti-inflammatory Approaches That Have Failed

G. J. del Zoppo

9.1 Introduction

Recent experimental work supports the thesis that inflammation is a pervasive and multifaceted accompaniment of focal brain ischemia. Whether it is a beneficial process meant to promote recovery and tissue healing, or detrimental, serving to increase an initially limited ischemic insult has been debated (del Zoppo et al. 2001). On the premise that both humoral and cellular inflammation contributes to tissue injury by promoting pan-necrosis or "neurodegeneration", defined as infarction in many small animal systems, a small number of anti-inflammatory approaches with therapeutic intent have been applied early to ischemic stroke patients in clinical trial.

The fundamental hypothesis tested by these studies is that humoral or cellular elements of inflammation contribute to the extension of early ischemic cerebral injury into irreversible injury. This treatise will consider some of the more readily discernible forces underlying the failure of recent clinical trials of agents that modulate inflammatory cell invasion in focal cerebral ischemia to demonstrate benefit (Table 1).

Table 1. Causes of stroke trial failures

Exacerbation of evolving CNS injury associated with focal ischemia
Failure to apply basic principles of immunology
Inadequate understanding of brain injury mechanisms
Exacerbation of systemic effects
Exacerbation of pre-existing infection or inflammatory condition
Failure to require an adequate experimental dataset
Failure to translate observations from phase II studies into phase III
Use of novel trial design elements not adequately tested
Failure to appreciate alternative hypotheses
Conflict of interest
Failure of the fundamental hypothesis

9.2 Experimental Basis for Cellular and Humoral Inflammation in Focal Cerebral Ischemia

The potential roles of inflammatory mediators in the evolution of ischemic cerebral injury have been examined in accepted models of middle cerebral artery occlusion (MCA:O) and forebrain (global) ischemia. Experimental work has suggested two related hypotheses: (a) polymorphonuclear (PMN) leukocytes participate in microvascular responses to ischemia, and (b) PMN leukocytes and other inflammatory cells contribute directly to brain tissue injury and neuronal death. PMN leukocytes can contribute to parenchymal injury by (a) causing additional impairment of local blood flow by microvessel obstruction, (b) exacerbating endothelial cell and matrix injury by releasing hydrolytic enzymes and generating oxygen free radicals, (c) initiating intravascular thrombus formation, and (d) emigrating into the ischemic parenchyma to potentially injure neurons and glial cells.

Hallenbeck and colleagues demonstrated the accumulation of ^{111}In-labeled autologous leukocytes in areas of low blood flow within 1–4 h after intra-arterial air embolism (Hallenbeck et al. 1986). Those observations were the first clear demonstration that PMN leukocytes could contribute to central nervous system (CNS) pathology in consequence of focal injury. Anderson et al. found correlations among the reduction in brain ATP content, the extent of neuronal injury, and the number of PMN leukocytes in the brain vessels and parenchyma following hypotension, and reperfusion to normotensive levels (Anderson et al. 1990). Hence, early work suggested that leukocytes could participate in cerebral injury.

Leukocyte invasion into the ischemic CNS involves (a) leukocyte activation, (b) altered microvascular reactivity and integrity, (c) microvessel obstruction, (d) leukocyte transmigration, and (e) the contributions of leukocyte-mediated phagocytosis to the evolving tissue injury. These events are modulated in part by the early recanalization of occluded cerebral arteries as demonstrated in experimental models and in atherothrombotic/embolic stroke in humans. Early recanalization can result in decreased infarct volume and improved neurologic outcome (del Zoppo et al. 1988, 1992a; Mori et al. 1988; Hacke et al. 1988; Mori et al. 1992b; The National Institutes of

Neurological Disorders and Stroke rt-PA Stroke Study Group 1995). Garcia and coworkers explored vascular and parenchymal alterations following permanent MCA:O in primates, cats, and Wistar rats (Garcia et al. 1977, 1983, 1993a,b; Zea-Longa et al. 1989). Subsequent studies indicated that PMN leukocytes rapidly enter the brain tissue in the ischemic territory (within 24 h in rodents), followed by the incursion of mononuclear cells (del Zoppo et al. 1991; Garcia et al. 1994). del Zoppo and colleagues examined the interplay of microvascular and parenchymal events following MCA:O/R in primates (del Zoppo et al. 1991, 1992b; Mori et al. 1992a; Thomas et al. 1993), while other groups subsequently explored a number of aspects of those observations (Zhang et al. 1994, 1995b, 1996, 1998; Chopp et al. 1994; Garcia et al. 1996). The initial steps in PMN leukocyte invasion of the ischemic cerebral territory following MCA:O involve the lodgement of PMN leukocytes in select capillaries and their firm adhesion to the endothelium of postcapillary venules (del Zoppo et al. 1991; Garcia et al. 1994).

Early studies of MCA:O in anesthetized primates did not identify microvessel occlusions in the ischemic territory, but intravascular thrombi were occasionally noted (Little et al. 1975, 1976). Carbon tracer techniques detected obstructions of presumed capillaries with periods of ischemia exceeding 3 h, which were attributed to "perivascular glial swelling and developing cerebral edema" (Little et al. 1975). However, in other experiments, microvessel occlusions were not observed in MCA:O time-course studies with anesthetized primates, although luminal encroachment by astrocyte swelling was identified (Garcia et al. 1983). The failure to find such obstructions early after MCA:O, particularly in light of the apparent loss of microvascular patency, could reflect a number of tissue preparation-related technical issues.

Ames et al. (Ames et al. 1968) and Fischer et al. (Fischer et al. 1977) attributed patchy loss of carbon tracer (the "no-reflow" phenomenon) in the cerebral hemispheres of rabbits undergoing transient global ischemia to microvascular events. Loss of microvessel patency after focal cerebral ischemia in an anesthetized primate MCA:O/R model was first suggested by Crowell et al. (Crowell et al. 1970; Crowell and Olsson 1972). Focal "no-reflow," under conditions of focal cerebral ischemia/reperfusion (I/R), was described by del Zoppo and colleagues in unanesthetized primates (Crowell et al. 1970; Crowell and Olsson 1972; Todd et al. 1986; del Zoppo et al. 1991; Mori et al. 1992a). The consistency of its appearance in non-human primate focal I/R preparations implies certain necessary conditions (del Zoppo et al. 1991; Barone et al. 1997). Similar findings have been made in rodents (Hamann et al. 2002). PMN leukocyte adhesion to the endothelium in postcapillary venules of the ischemic territory and their lodgement in capillaries by viscoelastic forces contributes in part to microvascular obstruction (Schmid-Schönbein 1987a; Garcia et al. 1993b, 1994; Okada et al. 1994b; Haring et al. 1996). In addition to intravascular cell-mediated microvascular flow obstruction, the no-reflow phenomenon has been attributed to extravascular compression (Garcia et al. 1983; Yoshida et al. 1992), intraluminal endothelial projections (Betz et al. 1994), endothelial cell swelling (del Zoppo et al. 1986), aggregated platelets (del Zoppo et al. 1991; Okada et al. 1994b), and fibrin formation (del Zoppo et al. 1991; Thomas et al. 1993).

Because of their large size (10–11 micron-diameter) and their viscoelastic properties, PMN leukocytes have restricted movement through the capillary portions of microvascular beds (Schmid-Schönbein 1987b, 1990, 1991). Recent studies of PMN leukocyte movement through the rat pial circulation indicate that, in the absence of ischemia, few PMN leukocytes roll along venular segments after moving through the capillary bed (Abels et al. 1994). However, PMN leukocytes do interact with cerebral microvessel endothelium in areas of injury (Härtl et al. 1996). Indeed, Mori et al. demonstrated that focal no-reflow could be significantly prevented by blockade of PMN leukocyte adhesion to activated endothelium using pharmacologic grade murine antihuman monoclonal antibody (MoAb) IB4 (60.3) to the granulocyte β_2-integrin CD18, infused before reperfusion (Mori et al. 1992a). Within the ischemic regions, degranulated platelets and fibrin also appear in close juxtaposition to PMN leukocytes within obstructed capillaries and larger noncapillary microvessels (del Zoppo et al. 1991). Fibrin deposition has also been documented within the vascular wall and lumina of capillaries within the ischemic zones, independent of leukocyte adhesion (Okada et al. 1994a). Hence, postischemic microvascular obstruction is a complex product of leukocyte dynamics and local activation of hemostasis.

Another interpretation of those observations is that leukocytes may be trapped in the ischemic regions (Garcia et al. 1994; Härtl et al. 1996). The low density of microvessels (<15%) displaying leukocyte adhesion receptors or adherent cells following MCA:O at any one time suggests the alternative concept that within the subcortex obstructed microvessels are bounded by those with cellular/plasma flow. Here, it could be hypothesized that local no-reflow can incorporate normal vessels with flow into an enlarging injury zone by secondary mechanisms [including inflammatory cell invasion (Tagaya et al. 2001)].

The initial movement of inflammatory cells into the ischemic CNS coincides with the appearance of the leukocyte adhesion receptors P-selectin, ICAM-1, and E-selectin on microvessel endothelium, together with their counterreceptors (e.g., PSGL-1, the β_2-integrin CD18 group) on leukocytes (Mori et al. 1992a; Okada et al. 1994b; Haring et al. 1996). P-selectin appears on the endothelium by 2 h MCA:O, followed by ICAM-1 by 4 h, and E-selectin between 7 and 24 h following MCA:O (during reperfusion) in the ischemic regions of the awake nonhuman primate (Okada et al. 1994b; Haring et al. 1996). Nonplatelet P-selectin is detectable on 5.5%–9.5% of microvessels throughout 24 h post-MCA:O (Garcia et al. 1993b), which could be explained by continued local thrombin generation (Roberts 1992). In contrast, ICAM-1 appeared maximally on $10.0 \pm 6.8\%$ of (noncapillary) microvessels at 4 h after MCA:O (Kawamura et al. 1990). E-selectin upregulation in the same territory was delayed, and marked by the appearance of the receptor on microvessels in the contralateral nonischemic hemisphere by 24 h following MCA:O (Haring et al. 1996). Both P- and E-selectin expression following MCA:O occurred only on microvessels with an intact basal lamina (Okada et al. 1994b; Haring et al. 1996). Similar observations have been made in rodent models of focal cerebral ischemia that indicate that these receptors appear simultaneously (Zhang et al. 1994, 1995b, 1998).

The cytokines, tumor neurosis factor (TNF-α) and interleukin-1 (IL-1β) are expressed in ischemic brain and influence the early progression of the inflammatory injury (Ginsberg and Myers 1972; Dawon et al. 1996; Barone and Feuerstein 1999; Shohami et al. 1999; Jander et al. 2000; Boutin et al. 2001). Both TNF-α and IL-1β

convert the luminal surface of endothelium from an antithrombotic and anti-inflammatory interface to a surface that is prothrombotic and proinflammatory (Hallenbeck 1996; Pober and Cotran 1999; Ruetzler et al. 2001). These proinflammatory cytokines can be produced by endothelial cells (Gourin and Shackford 1997), perivascular macrophages (Woodroofe and Cuzner 1993; Buttini et al. 1994), microglia (Buttini et al. 1996), astrocytes (Lieberman et al. 1989), and neurons (Saito et al. 1996; Gourin and Shackford 1997; Davies et al. 1999). Following brain ischemia, IL-1β increases within 3–6 h and peaks between 3–5 days (Saito et al. 1996; Legos et al. 2000), while TNF-α appears within 0.5–1 h after ischemia and peaks at 8–24 h, with a substantial decline by 4 days (Liu et al. 1994; Buttini et al. 1996). IL-1β and TNF-α can affect microglia, astrocytes, and neurons through signaling mediated by their receptors, the IL-1 receptor I, the TNF-α receptor 1, and the TNF-α receptor 2 (Botchkina et al. 1997; Touzani et al. 1999).

IL-1β has been clearly implicated in the progression of ischemic brain injury (Boutin et al. 2001). Administration of IL-1β directly into ischemic brain exacerbates damage in stroke models. Injection or overexpression of the interleukin-1 receptor antagonist IL-1ra, the natural IL-1β inhibitor, or blockade of IL-1β converting enzyme activity, reduces infarction volumes in preclinical stroke models (Graveland and DiFiglia 1985; Loddick et al. 1997; Rothwell et al. 1997). There is also evidence that TNF-α contributes to ischemic brain damage (Shohami et al. 1999). Inhibition with the recombinant type 1 soluble TNF receptor, TNF binding protein (TNFbp), significantly reduced the impairment of microvascular perfusion in the ischemic injury zone and reduced infarct volume in experimental focal brain ischemia (Dawon et al. 1996). Several groups have also demonstrated cytoprotection by TNFbp or neutralizing anti-TNF antibodies in preclinical stroke models (Barone et al. 1997; Meistrell et al. 1997; Nawashiro et al. 1997a; Yang et al. 1998).

However, the observed effects of IL-1β and TNF-α in injured brain have not been uniformly cytotoxic (Strijbos and Rothwell 1995; Ohtsuki et al. 1996; Tasaki et al. 1997; Nawashiro et al. 1997b; Liu et al. 2000). These inflammatory cytokines may function as mediators of a sublethal "preconditioning" stress that induce protean adaptations to a subsequent potentially lethal stress rather than acting as direct neuroprotectants. More importantly, the available data provides strong support for a cytotoxic effect of the inflammatory cytokines as well as evidence to support a neuroprotective role for these intercellular signaling molecules (Bruce et al. 1996; Boutin et al. 2001). This suggests that knowing the precise timing and targets of these cytokines could be important for inhibiting their action in the clinical setting. Alternatively, the multifaceted nature of their activities in the CNS may limit the clinical success of any inhibitory strategy.

Leukocyte transmigration in the CNS occurs at both interendothelial tight junctions and through endothelial cells. Activated leukocytes have been detected as early as 1 h after MCA:O on the abluminal side of select microvessels (Abumiya et al. 1999). Dereski et al. noted the appearance of PMN leukocytes in both the vascular and parenchymal compartments from several minutes up to 8 h after MCA:O, reaching a maximum at 72 h in anesthetized Wistar rats (Dereski et al. 1992). Transmigration across postcapillary venules began 4–6 h after MCA occlusion, with maximum invasion into the ischemic parenchyma by 24 h after MCA occlusion (Garcia et al. 1993a). Coagulation necrosis was apparent in the ischemic area 24–48 h after MCA:O (Garcia et al. 1993a). Those observations were supported by the appearance of granulocytes into the ischemic zone within 30 min of proximal MCA:O (Zea-Longa et al. 1989; Garcia et al. 1993b, 1994). They suggest a temporal sequence of PMN leukocyte invasion followed by neuronal necrosis. However, it is yet unclear whether the two biological phenomena are causally related.

Evidence for leukocyte adhesion in the pial microvasculature during focal ischemia (which affects the cortical tissue) is conflicting (Heinel et al. 1994; Härtl et al. 1996; Ritter et al. 2000). Abels and coworkers did not observe an increase in the number of PMN leukocytes that roll in the pial vasculature after brief carotid occlusion and reperfusion in a rat model of MCA territory ischemia (Abels et al. 1994). Environmental risks, particularly those that can stimulate PMN leukocyte activation and rolling (e.g., products of cigarette incineration) find effect in the superficial vasculature (von Adrian et al. 1991; Lehr et al. 1993). In sum, leukocytes appear in the territory of focal ischemia, and probably contribute to the ultimate injury (infarction).

During this evolution of injury, extracellular matrix (ECM) components of the vascular basal lamina (laminin-1, laminin-5, collagen IV, and fibronectin) disappear together (Hamann et al. 1995, 1996). One explanation for their disappearance during MCA:O/R may be proteolysis from endogenous sources of proteases secreted by vascular cells including MMPs and plasminogen activators (Levin and del Zoppo 1994; Krane 1994; Rosenberg et al. 1996; Clark et al. 1997; Fujimura et al. 1999; Heo et al. 1999; Hosomi et al. 2001), or from the release of PMN leukocyte granule enzymes, which include collagenase (MMP-8), gelatinase (MMP-9), elastase, and cathepsin G during the inflammatory phase following ischemia (Murphy et al. 1987; Pike et al. 1989; Watanabe et al. 1990; Heck et al. 1990; Krane 1994).

More direct support for a CNS tissue-damaging role for leukocytes comes from observations in murine transgenic models in which the genes for P-selectin, ICAM-1, or NADPH oxidase have been deleted (Soriano et al. 1996; Connolly et al. 1997; Walder et al. 1997). In the murine NADPH oxidase $^{(-/-)}$ constructs, the phagocyte oxidase is absent, so that the respiratory burst does not occur, specifically impairing PMN leukocyte-medicated tissue injury (Walder et al. 1997). The decrease in injury with this construct is significant. Studies with P-selectin $^{(-/-)}$ and ICAM-1 $^{(-/-)}$ constructs, which display reduced expression of the respective leukocyte adhesion receptors, indicate the cytotoxic effects of leukocyte-endothelial cell interactions in ischemia-induced inflammation (Soriano et al. 1996; Connolly et al. 1997).

Numerous experiments have suggested that altered PMN leukocyte function or induced leukopenia can improve defined responses to cerebrovascular obstruction (reperfusion), including edema formation, neuronal injury, infarction volume, and neurologic outcome in preclinical models. Strategies that block granulocyte adhesion can decrease transmigration of PMN leukocytes and edema formation. Bednar et al. documented a substantial decrease in edema formation after using an anti-CD18 MoAb in a rabbit multivessel occlusion/hypotension model of focal cerebral ischemia (Bednar et al. 1992). Those results can be explained by the abrogation of granulocyte adhesion to the postcapillary venule endothelium, reduced endothelial permeability, and decreased PMN leukocyte egress, in keeping with the known interactions between activated granulocytes and venule endothelium (Kuroiwa et al. 1985). In separate experiments, cerebral infarct volume was reduced by a polyclonal antineutrophil serum given before the onset of focal/hemispheric ischemia in a complex rabbit model of thromboembolism/induced hypotension (Bednar et al. 1991). Vasthare et al. demonstrated that leukopenia induced in a rodent carotid artery ligation model of reversible forebrain ischemia was accompanied by preservation of electroencephalographic activity and evoked potential peak amplitude (Vasthare et al. 1990; Heinel et al. 1994).

Blockade of the leukocyte β_2-integrin CD18 following MCA:O and prior to reperfusion significantly increased microvascular patency in postcapillary venules relative to control (Mori et al. 1992a). Similarly, specific inhibitors of the platelet integrin $\alpha_{IIb}\beta_3$-fibrin receptor reduced microvascular no-reflow in the nonhuman primate (Abumiya et al. 2000) and injury volume in the mouse (Coudhri et al. 1998). Those studies support the contribution of leukocytes and platelets to postcapillary venular occlusion. Antileukocyte strategies which can decrease injury have included the antineutrophil antibody RP-3 and antibodies against leukocyte CD11b and CD18, or endothelial cell ICAM-1 (Matsuo et al. 1994; Chopp et al. 1994; Zhang et al. 1995b). Kogure and colleagues described a beneficial effect of leukopenia on edema formation and infarct volume after focal cerebral I/R in a well-characterized experimental model (Matsuo et al. 1994). Many of the leukocyte inhibition studies have shown reductions in injury volume ranging from about 30% to 60%. However, there are also negative studies. Härtl et al. have examined some of those studies critically (Härtl et al. 1996). In general, both the gene deletion and interventional experiments support the concept that activated PMN leukocytes can contribute to the evolution of permanent tissue injury during ischemic stroke.

9.3 Clinical Evidence for Inflammation Accompanying Ischemic Stroke

Inflammation plays a central role in tissue wound recovery and repair, as a part of the host immune defense system. Occlusion of a

brain-supplying artery initiates responses in the downstream microvasculature and the surrounding ischemic tissue, which stimulate
leukocyte invasion and accumulation, cellular activation, and neuronal and glial necrosis, which suggest wound recovery. These responses involve the rapid appearance of specific transcription factors
(e.g., NF-κB), the release of cytokines and chemokines, activation of
microvascular endothelial cells and leukocytes, the generation of re-
ciprocal adhesion receptors, leukocyte transmigration, and changes
in microvessel perfusion and integrity. These elements of "secondary
injury" of the CNS are discerned nearly exclusively from experimental studies.

However, leukocyte-containing infiltrates have been observed in
the ischemic areas of cerebral tissues from patients succumbing
from ischemic stroke (Zülch and Kleihues 1966; Adams and Sidman
1968; Okazaki 1983; Moossy 1985; Graham 1992). Postmortem
studies suggest that after 24 h, leukocytes are abundant at the edge
of an ischemic lesion, but are rare in the central region (Graham
1992). Between 24 and 36 h, PMN leukocytes appear around small
blood vessels and throughout the entire infarct (Adams and Sidman
1968). Zülch noted that leukocytes (not otherwise characterized)
emigrate diffusely from veins about 16 h after the injury following
experimental brain embolism in cats (Zülch and Kleihues 1966). On
the premise that leukocyte transmigration contributes to the evolution of pannecrosis of the ischemic territory, four clinical trials testing distinct inhibitors of endothelial cell-leukocyte adhesion or chemotaxis have been undertaken. Their general design characteristics
and outcomes as far as they are known are summarized here.

9.3.1 The Enlimomab Acute Stroke Trial:
Inhibition of Endothelial Cell ICAM-1

An anti-ICAM-1 MoAb, R6.5 (a murine IgG_{2a} MoAb), under development as an antileukocyte adhesion strategy was applied in the
acute setting of ischemic stroke. Impetus for the clinical development of Enlimomab was attributed to preclinical studies using other
anti-ICAM-1 strategies (Clark et al. 1991; Bowes et al. 1993; Zhang
et al. 1994, 1995a). The pharmokinetics and safety of Enlimomab

were tested in an open label phase II dose-finding study in 32 patients hospitalized with the diagnosis of stroke (Schneider et al. 1998). Target serum levels of Enlimomab were achieved in all patients in the higher dose-rates. Adverse events occurred in 14 patients (including pneumonia, sepsis, cardiac failure, and cardiac arrest), but a single serious adverse event occurred when a patient suffered an anaphylactic reaction from receiving an unfiltered load of the antibody. Mortality was not increased by exposure to Enlimomab in that study (Schneider et al. 1998). Based upon that experience, a phase III trial was undertaken which randomized 625 patients presenting with ischemic stroke to placebo ($n=308$) or Enlimomab ($n=317$) within 6 h from symptom onset (Enlimomab Acute Stroke Trial Investigators 2003). The murine antibody was infused over 5 consecutive days by single infusion each day. After baseline assessment, patients were then evaluated on days 5 and 90 after initiation of treatment. At day 90, the modified Rankin Scale (mRS) score was significantly worse in those who received Enlimomab compared to those receiving placebo. In addition, fewer patients displayed symptom-free recovery who had received Enlimomab than placebo, and mortality was significantly greater. There were significantly greater adverse events with Enlimomab than placebo, primarily consisting of infection and fever (Enlimomab Acute Stroke Trial Investigators 2003). Although patients who had experienced fever were more likely to have a poor outcome or die, there was no clear relationship to the test agent. A relationship between the infusion of Enlimomab over 5 days and the significantly poorer outcome of patients receiving this agent has been sought.

Two additional observations are relevant to the phase III trial outcomes. A recent study in an established rat stroke model employing a much used murine antibody directed against rat ICAM-1 (1A29), when infused twice prior to MCA:O induced rat antimouse antibodies, and activated complement, PMN leukocytes, and the vascular endothelium (Furuya et al. 2001). That approach, which mimicked the clinical trial of Enlimomab, overwhelmed any potential benefit from inhibition of leukocyte accumulation, and increased infarct volume. That study suggested that single or multiple exposures to intravenously administered heterologous proteins might activate local inflammatory mechanisms which increase ischemic brain injury. In addition, after completion of the Enlimomab trial it was demonstrated that R6.5 could promote leukocyte activation (Vuorte et al. 1999).

9.3.2 The HALT Stroke Study: An Anti-leukocyte Adhesion Strategy

A second antileukocyte adhesion strategy employed a humanized murine MoAb against the leukocyte β_2-integrin CD18 (Hu23F2G), in patients with symptoms of ischemic stroke. Patients were acquired within 12 h of symptom onset, and had a baseline NIHSS score of 4–22. The phase II double blind placebo-controlled dose-rate finding safety study was conducted simultaneously with a preclinical study testing the effects of Hu23F2G on a rabbit model of transient focal ischemia (Yenari et al. 1998). A significant reduction in PMN leukocyte infiltration and in the region of ischemic damage was noted among those animals receiving Hu23F2G ($n=8$) over placebo ($n=7$; Yenari et al. 1998). That study was consistent with others suggesting a central role for leukocytes in the evolution of the ischemic lesion.

The clinical experience, now in the public domain, was that Hu23F2G did not significantly negatively affect mortality compared to placebo within the 12-h window in the phase II study. Furthermore, no difference in mortality was noted in that study. Based upon the favorable safety profile, a phase III three-arm placebo-controlled trial, enrolling patients within 12 h of symptom onset was undertaken. Patients also could receive rt-PA within the NINDS protocol guidelines. Two Hu23F2G dose regimens (which involved a single dose on enrollment, or a dose of Hu23F2G both at time of enrollment and 60 h later) where compared with placebo. That trial was not completed as planned, but was terminated at the first interim assessment when a futility analysis suggested that no benefit of the treatment would occur even if the study was continued (ICOS Stroke Trial 2000). To date, no public information is available regarding the outcomes, safety issues, or the relative number of serious adverse events in that phase III trial.

9.3.3 Recombinant Neutrophil Inhibitory Factor (rNIF): An Anti-leukocyte Transmigration Strategy

A phase II study of recombinant neutrophil inhibitory factor (rNIF; UK279, 276) was undertaken to test the hypothesis that a novel inhibitor of neutrophil transmigration could reduce injury and morbidity from ischemic stroke if applied in the acute setting. rNIF is a novel 41-kDa glycoprotein β_2-integrin (CD18) antagonist, derived from a hookworm. Functional interaction between rNIF and domain I of CD11b/CD18 has been described (Muchowski et al. 1994). Published preclinical work-up in experimental focal CNS injury determined a dose-response of infarction volume after permanent MCA:O and transient focal ischemia (Jiang et al. 1995, 1998). It was claimed that continuous infusion for 6 h was insufficient to demonstrate an effect on the final injury volume; however, continuous infusion for 48 h or 7 days could reduce infarction volume (Jiang et al. 1995, 1998).

The clinical phase II dose-finding study in patients was predicated upon a Bayesian approach: patients were placed in "open" dose–rate cohorts depending upon the experience of previously treated patients in other dose-rate groups in the prospective safety study. Acceptable outcomes included improvement in mRS at 30 and 90 days. A recent presentation of the study outcome data indicated that the trial had failed to demonstrate a dose–effect. No phase III study has been undertaken so far.

9.3.4 Trial of Interleukin-1 Receptor Antagonist (IL-1ra): A Strategy to Inhibit Cytokine Activity

A prospective phase II placebo-controlled study of the cytokine antagonist recombinant IL-1ra in patients with ischemic stroke who are acquired within 12 h of symptom onset is underway in the UK at a limited number of sites. Given the favorable safety profile of IL-1ra as an anti-inflammatory agent in arthritic disorders and in rodent models of focal cerebral ischemia, no adverse safety effects have been expected (Graveland and DiFiglia 1985; Loddick et al. 1997; Rothwell et al. 1997). The phase II study has not yet been completed, and no data are available for assessment at this writing.

9.4 Possible Limitations to Clinical Trial Success

A balanced view of the clinical trial experience with the novel anti-inflammatory agents so far applied in the setting of ischemic stroke is that the fundamental hypothesis that blockade of cellular inflammation will reduce the ultimate CNS lesion following focal ischemia has not been disproved. Neither has it been proven. One personal view is that the hypothesis has not been adequately tested owing in part to (a) technical inadequacies in the several trials, (b) specific limitations in trial design, and/or (c) limitations in the experimental run-up to those trials. The following are some general concerns raised by the clinical trial experience with these anti-inflammatory approaches. It should be noted that all agents tested so far are biologicals derived from mammalian sources or cell lines.

9.4.1 The Intervention Exacerbated Evolving CNS Injury Associated with Focal Ischemia

The premise here is that the intervention, either directly or via pathways activated upon exposure of the brain to the test agent, resulted in an acceleration or the extension of the injury initiated by ischemia. Activation of circulating blood cells (e.g., monocytes or PMN leukocytes), complement, or induction of microvascular thrombosis could indirectly provide contributions to the evolving injury. Exposure of the injured neuropil to the test agent or to inflammatory cells activated by exposure to the test agent could exacerbate the injury, because of penetration of the agent or its factors through the permeable microvessel blood brain barrier. An example of this condition is the phase III study of Enlimomab. This situation could have been avoided by appropriate preclinical studies to test this premise.

9.4.2 Failure to Apply Basic Principles of Immunology

The serial infusion of heterologous antibodies or humanized test agents is highly likely to activate complement, activate the immune system, and/or generate antiagent antibodies. Little is known about the effect of these elements on the evolving injury of the ischemic brain. But, it is likely to be deleterious. It has been proposed that human antimurine antibodies were generated during the five-day infusion of Enlimomab. Detectable effects of these autologous antibodies on cells of the monocytoid lineage would be expected to occur. Activation of complement, generation of activated lymphocyte subsets, and other effects are likely. A recent experimental study by Furuya et al. reproduced portions of this clinical experiment, and demonstrated that serial infusion (into rats) of a heterologous (murine) antibody raised against the rat endothelial cell leukocyte receptor ICAM-1 could increase behavioral disability and demise compared to controls (Furuya et al. 2001). Activation of cell-signaling mechanisms (e.g., endothelial cell, or glial cell) could hypothetically exacerbate injury. This notion has not been tested adequately in the CNS, but is known from interventions in the circulating blood (e.g., binding of receptor activable antibodies). An implication for the effects of receptor blockade on outcome is that they may depend upon the type of injury and the intactness of the microvascular barrier.

9.4.3 Inadequate Understanding of Brain Injury Mechanisms

While elements important for cellular inflammation have been described in experimental models (e.g., the cytokines IL-1β and TNF-α, and select chemokines), those triggering elements stimulated by ischemia that are necessary for the expression and secretion of agonists for inflammation are largely unknown, as are their cell sources. Complement expression and activation is largely unexplored, in part because of intrinsic limitations of complement biology in experimental models. Furthermore, events which lead to ultimate infarction are not likely to reflect the very early (i.e., within hours) postischemic events. The stimuli which might modulate these events, both early and late, are yet to be elucidated.

9.4.4 Exacerbation of Systemic Effects

Here, promotion of inflammation and/or complement activation would be expected to exacerbate systemic processes which may have a secondary effect on the brain responses to injury. The notion that hyperpyrexia could cause increased injury falls into this category. Initial concerns that the deleterious effects of Enlimomab may have been due to the induction of fever (and the latter's effect on CNS function following ischemia) have proved specious. However, this concern could be generalized to the phase II studies of Hu23F2G, rNIF, and IL-1ra (ongoing). There has been no specific indication that fever was induced in the early moments of ischemic stroke by these agents, however. But, this conclusion also reflects the limited information available from those studies.

9.4.5 Exacerbation of Pre-existing Infection or Inflammatory Conditions

Evidence exists that inhibition of leukocyte adhesion may exacerbate pre-existing infections (e.g., intravenous catheter site infections, urinary tract infections) that are not attended by antibiotics. Early recognition and adequate medical treatment significantly reduces these potential adverse events. Their frequency has been a concern of all trials so far, although their impact on these trials has been uncertain.

9.4.6 Failure to Require an Adequate Dataset to Translate Experimental Outcomes to Clinical Trial Design

Concern can be raised when a single laboratory or a single experimental setting (e.g., a single species) is employed as a prelude for a large phase II or III study. While preclinical work supported the clinical studies of rNIF, Hu23F2G, and Enlimomab, concerns regarding the adequacy and appropriateness of those datasets have been raised retrospectively. Careful consideration of the development program suggests that the clinical trial undertaking and experimental science were often not connected.

9.4.7 Failure to Translate Observations from Phase II Studies into Phase III Trials

There is little evidence that the extrapolated positive effects of efficacy projected from the phase II safety study data have been reproduced by an adequately powered phase III trial of the test agent in early ischemic stroke. This implies an inability to reproduce the study conditions of the phase II trial, inappropriateness of the extrapolation, or inactivity of the agent. The most sensitive and under-appreciated element in this translation is the nature of the patient population. It could suffer from scale-up, pressures to complete a trial by a prespecified due date, or the use of the same investigators/centers that have previously served negative trials. Inadequate insight into the failures of those trials would then be compounded in new trials. One approach to this growing problem is to identify "active" subgroups within the study population. Another is to generate a better understanding of CNS injury response mechanisms.

9.4.8 Use of Novel Trial Design Elements Not Previously or Adequately Tested

The evaluation of the efficacy of rNIF in early ischemic stroke in a phase II safety/efficacy study employed a scheme of patient acquisition based upon Bayesian analysis. Both the putatively active agent and the analytic system were untried for this setting. Furthermore, very limited preclinical experimentation with the compound was available with which to guide the clinical trial design. Hence three elements were potentially compromised in that test. In contrast, in the phase II portion of PROACT, in which a novel delivery system and agent were tested (i.e., direct infusion single chain urokinase), a significant contribution of heparin to increased recanalization efficacy and intracerebral hemorrhage was suspected during the trial. An adjustment of the heparin dose was undertaken when an excess of hemorrhage was suspected (del Zoppo et al. 1998). The consequence was a readjustment of both recanalization frequency and hemorrhage in the direction of safety. That is an example of a small study group for which study design adjustment could be readily made.

9.4.9 Failure to Appreciate Alternative Hypotheses

In the Enlimomab study, the possibility of enhanced cerebral injury caused by the anti-inflammatory agent was not appreciated (see Sect. 9.4.1). In a separate setting, futility analyses performed early in a trial of limited size (e.g., the Hu23F2G phase III trial) would be likely to underestimate the efficacy effect, and thereby underpower the conclusions. Here data are lacking to prove the alternative as the dataset has not been made public. On the other hand, an apparently robustly powered study (e.g., the rNIF phase II trial) could fail if the presumed effect of the agent and the outcome(s) to be measured do not have a predictable relationship, or there is no relationship. This is a particular difficulty when the phase III study tests a principle, outcome measure, or hypothesis with an agent that has unproven relevance to the hypothesis, test strategy, or outcome. Then many alternative hypotheses are possible.

9.4.10 Conflict of Interest

Settings in which investigators have a stake in the trial design and in the commercial benefits from conduct of the trial are unacceptable, and challenge the veracity of the study. This is particularly so when the investigator can potentially realize material gain. Here, study design or conduct can suffer, and a balanced interpretation of the outcome may not be forthcoming. The impact on future trials can be chilling.

9.4.11 Failure of the Fundamental Hypothesis

In view of obvious technical and design limitations that have contributed significantly to the failure of clinical trials of the three anti-inflammatory approaches so far tested, it cannot be excluded that the primary hypothesis is appropriate. Indeed, the bulk of experimental evidence so far and the impressions from the clinical setting of ischemic stroke support the fundamental hypothesis. Refinements of the hypothesis that must be considered relate to timing of the interventions, systemic effects of those interventions, the biochemical structure of the anti-inflammatory agents to be tested, the target patient subpopulations, and the nature of CNS responses to injury. Furthermore, given the multifaceted nature of inflammatory stimuli it is not certain whether blockade of a single specific site would have detectable clinical effects.

9.5 Conclusions

While there is substantial evidence that focal ischemia of the cerebral tissues can initiate an inflammatory response, and that both cellular and humoral inflammation comprise part of the secondary response to ischemia, three of the four clinical trials so far undertaken with inhibitors of cellular inflammation (e.g., Enlimomab, Hu23F2G, and rNIF) have not shown efficacy in the studies in which they were used. Those trials have been limited in scope, and have several notable shortcomings in concept or design. Whether inhibition of a single or of multiple steps in the inflammatory response to ischemia could be successfully detected depends upon the development of sensitive and relevant outcome measures. Furthermore, experience so far suggests that ischemic brain tissue exposed to heterologous agents or activated cells can display enhanced injury. This is an important observation, but also emphasizes the paucity of information yet available about the evolution of cerebral injury and the limitations that current animal models provide. Nonetheless, understanding the manner in which brain injury evolves requires testing in animal models. In view of the observation that the fundamental hypothesis has not been adequately or appropriately tested, as recently stated, it is critical that both well-designed experimental and clinical studies of anti-inflammatory approaches to ischemic stroke proceed (del Zoppo et al. 2001).

Acknowledgements. This work was supported in part by grants R01 NS26945 and R01 NS38710 of the National Institutes of Health. Portions of the manuscript were previously developed as a chapter with Dr. John Hallenbeck. Thanks are expressed to Michael Piellucci for his contributions to this manuscript.

References

Abels C, Röhrich F, Uhl E, Corvin S, Villringer A, Dirnagl U, Baethmann A, Schürer L (1994) Current evidence on a pathophysiological of leukocyte/endothelial interactions in cerebral ischemia. In: Hartmann A, Yatsu F, Kuschinsky W (eds) Brain ischemia and basic mechanisms. Springer, Heidelberg, pp 366–372

Abumiya T, Lucero J, Heo JH, Tagaya M, Koziol JA, Copeland BR, del Zoppo GJ (1999) Activated microvessels express vascular endothelial growth factor and integrin $a_v\beta_3$ during focal cerebral ischemia. J Cereb Blood Flow Metab 19:1038–1050

Abumiya T, Fitridge R, Mazur C, Copeland BR, Koziol JA, Tschopp JF, Pierschbacher MD, del Zoppo GJ (2000) Integrin $a_{IIb}\beta_3$ inhibitor preserves microvascular patency in experimental acute focal cerebral ischemia. Stroke 31:1402–1410

Adams RD, Sidman RL (1968) Cerebrovascular disease. In: Adams RD, Sidman RL (eds) Introduction to neuropathology. McGraw-Hill, New York, pp 171–183

Ames A, III, Wright RC, Kowada M, Thurston JM, Majno G (1968) Cerebral ischemia. The nonreflow phenomenon. Am J Pathol 52:437–453

Anderson ML, Smith DS, Nioka S, Subramanian H, Garcia JH, Halsey JH, Chance B (1990) Experimental brain ischemia: assessment of injury by magnetic resonance spectroscopy and histology. Neurol Res 12:195–204

Barone FC, Feuerstein GZ (1999) Inflammatory mediators and stroke: new opportunities for novel therapeutics. J Cereb Blood Flow Metab 19:819–834

Barone FC, Arvin B, White RF, Miller A, Webb CL, Willette RN, Lysko PG, Feuerstein GZ (1997) Tumor necrosis factor: a mediator of focal ischemic brain injury. Stroke 28:1233–1244

Bednar MM, Raymond S, McAuliffe T, Lodge PA, Gross CE (1991) The role of neutrophils and platelets in a rabbit model of thromboembolic stroke. Stroke 22:44–50

Bednar MM, Gross CE, Raymond S, Wright SD, Kohut JJ (1992) IB4, a monoclonal antibody against the CD18 adhesion complex of leukocytes, attenuates intracranial hypertension in a rabbit stroke model. Stroke 23:152

Betz AL, Keep RF, Beer ME, Ren XD (1994) Blood-brain permeability and brain concentration of sodium, potassium, and chloride during focal ischemia. J Cereb Blood Flow Metab 14:29–37

Botchkina GI, Meistrell ME, Botchkina IL, Tracey KJ (1997) Expression of TNF and TNF receptors (p55 and p75) in the rat brain after focal cerebral ischemia. Mol Med 3:765–781

Boutin H, LeFeuvre RA, Horai R, Asano M, Iwakura Y, Rothwell NJ (2001) Role of IL-1a and IL-1β in ischemic brain damage. J Neurosci 21:5528–5534

Bowes MP, Zivin JA, Rothlein R (1993) Monoclonal antibody to the ICAM-1 adhesion site reduces neurological damage in a rabbit cerebral embolism stroke model. Exp Neurol 119:215–219

Bruce AJ, Boling W, Kindy MS, Peschon J, Kraemer PJ, Carpenter MK, Holtsberg FW, Mattson MP (1996) Altered neuronal and microglial responses to excitotoxic and ischemic brain injury in mice lacking TNF receptors. Nat Med 2:788–794

Buttini M, Sauter A, Boddeke HW (1994) Induction of interleukin-1β mRN after focal cerebral ischaemia in the rat. Mol Brain Res 23:126–134

Buttini M, Appel K, Sauter A, Gebicke-Haerter PJ, Boddeke HWGM (1996) Expression of tumor necrosis factor a after focal cerebral ischaemia in the rat. Neuroscience 71:1–16

Chopp M, Zhang RL, Chen H, Li Y, Jiang N, Rusche JR (1994) Post-ischemic administration of an anti-Mac-1 antibody reduces ischemic cell damage after transient middle cerebral artery occlusion in rats. Stroke 25:869–875

Clark AW, Krekoski CA, Bou Shao-Sun, Chapman KR, Edwards DR (1997) Increased gelatinase A (MMP-2) and gelatinase B (MMP-9) activities in human brain after focal ischemia. Neurosci Lett 238:53–56

Clark WM, Madden KP, Rothlein R, Zivin JA (1991) Reduction of central nervous system ischemic injury by monoclonal antibody to intercellular adhesion molecule. J Neurosurg 75:623–627

Connolly Jr ES, Winfree CJ, Prestigiacomo CJ, Kim SC, Choudri TF, Hoh BL, Naka Y, Solomon RA, Pinsky DJ (1997) Exacerbation of cerebral injury in mice that express the P-selectin gene: identification of P-selectin blockade as a new target for the treatment of stroke. Circ Res 81:304–310

Coudhri TF, Hoh BL, Zerwes HG, Prestigiacomo CJ, Kim SC, Connolly E, Sander Jr E, Kottirsch G, Pinsky DJ (1998) Reduced microvascular thrombosis and improved outcome in acute murine stroke by inhibiting GP IIb/IIIa receptor-mediated platelet aggregation. J Clin Invest 102:1301–1310

Crowell RM, Olsson Y (1972) Impaired microvascular filling after focal cerebral ischemia in the monkey. Neurology 22:500–504

Crowell RM, Olsson Y, Klatzo I, Ommaya A (1970) Temporary occlusion of the middle cerebral artery in monkeys. Clinical and pathological observations. Stroke 1:439–448

Davies CA, Loddick SA, Toulmond S, Stroemer RP, Hunt J, Rothwell NJ (1999) The progression and topographic distribution of interleukin-1 expression after permanent middle cerebral artery occlusion in the rat. J Cereb Blood Flow Metab 19:87–98

Dawon DA, Martin D, Hallenbeck JM (1996) Inhibition of tumor necrosis factor-a reduces focal cerebral ischemic injury in the spontaneously hypertensive rat. Neuroscience Lett 218:41–44 del Zoppo GJ, Copeland BR, Harker LA, Waltz TA, Zyroff J, Hanson SR, Battenberg E (1986) Experimental acute thrombotic stroke in baboons. Stroke 17:1254–1265

del Zoppo GJ, Ferbert A, Otis S, Brückmann H, Hacke W, Zyroff J, Harker LA, Zeumer H (1988) Local intra-arterial fibrinolytic therapy in acute carotid territory stroke: a pilot study. Stroke 19:307–313

del Zoppo GJ, Schmid-Schönbein GW, Mori E, Copeland BR, Chang C-M (1991) Polymorphonuclear leukocytes occlude capillaries following middle cerebral artery occlusion and reperfusion in baboons. Stroke 22: 1276–1284

del Zoppo GJ, Poeck K, Pessin MS, Wolpert SM, Furlan AJ, Ferbert A, Alberts MJ, Zivin JA, Wechsler L, Busse O, Greenlee Jr R, Brass L, Mohr JP, Feldmann E, Hacke W, Kase CS, Biller J, Gress D, Otis SM (1992a) Recombinant tissue plasminogen activator in acute thrombotic and embolic stroke. Ann Neurol 32:78–86

del Zoppo GJ, Yu J-Q, Copeland BR, Thomas WS, Schneiderman J, Morrissey J (1992b) Tissue factor location in nonhuman primate cerebral tissue. Thromb Haemost 68:642–647

del Zoppo GJ, Higashida RT, Furlan AJ, Pessin MS, Rowley HA, Gent M, and the PROACT Investigators (1998) PROACT: A phase II randomized trial of recombinant prourokinase by direct arterial delivery in acute middle cerebral artery stroke. Stroke 29:4–11

del Zoppo GJ, Becker KJ, Hallenbeck JM (2001) Inflammation after stroke: is it harmful? Arch Neurol 58:669–672

Dereski MO, Chopp M, Knight RA, Chen H, Garcia JH (1992) Focal cerebral ischemia in the rat: Temporal profile of neutrophil responses. Neurosci Res Commun 11:179–186

Enlimomab Acute Stroke Trial Investigators (2003) Use of anti-ICAM-1 therapy in ischemic stroke: results of the Enlimomab Acute Stroke Trial. Neurology 57:1428–1434

Fischer EG, Ames A, Hedley-White ET, O'Gorman S (1977) Reassessment of cerebral capillary changes in acute global ischemia and their relationship to the "no-reflow phenomenon". Stroke 8:36–39

Fujimura M, Gasche Y, Morita-Fujimura Y, Massengale J, Kawase M, Chan PH (1999) Early appearance of activated matrix metalloproteinase-9 and blood-brain barrier disruption in mice after focal cerebral ischemia and reperfusion. Brain Res 842:92–100

Furuya K, Takeda H, Azhar S, McCarron RM, DeGraba TJ, Rothlein R, Hugli TE, del Zoppo GJ, Hallenback JM (2001) Examination of several potential mechanisms for the negative outcome in a clinical stroke trial of enlimomab, a murine antihuman ICAM-1 antibody. Stroke 32:2665–2674

Garcia JH, Kalimo H, Kamijyo Y (1977) Cellular events during partial cerebral ischemia. 1. Electron microscopy of feline cerebral cortex after middle cerebral artery occlusion. Virchows Arch [B] 25:191–206

Garcia JH, Mitchem HL, Briggs L, Morawetz R, Hudetz AG, Hazelrig JB, Halsey Jr JH, Conger KA (1983) Transient focal ischemia in subhuman primates: neuronal injury as a function of local cerebral blood flow. J Neuropathol Exp Neurol 42:44–60

Garcia JH, Yoshida Y, Chen H, Li Y, Zhang ZG, Liam J, Chen S, Chopp M (1993a) Progression from ischemic injury to infarct following middle cerebral artery occlusion in the rat. Am J Pathol 142:623–635

Garcia JH, Yoshida Y, Lian J, Chen S, Chen H, Li Y, Chopp M (1993b) Experimental occlusion of a middle cerebral artery (MCA) is accompanied by early polymorphonuclear leukocyte infiltration. Stroke 24:166

Garcia JH, Liu KF, Yoshida Y, Lian J, Chen S, del Zoppo GJ (1994) Influx of leukocytes and platelets in an evolving brain infarct (Wistar rat). Am J Pathol 144:188–199

Garcia JH, Liu K-F, Bree MP (1996) Effects of CD11b/18 monoclonal antibody on rats with permanent middle cerebral artery occlusion. Am J Pathol 148:241–248

Ginsberg MD, Myers RE (1972) The topography of impaired microvascular perfusion in the primate brain following total circulatory arrest. Neurology 22:998–1011

Gourin CG, Shackford SR (1997) Production of tumor necrosis factor A and interleukin-1 by human cerebral microvascular endothelium after percussive trauma. J Trauma 42:1101–1107

Graham DI (1992) Hypoxia and vascular disorders. In: Adams JH, Duchen LW (eds) Greenfield's neuropathology. Oxford University Press, New York, pp 198–200

Graveland GA, DiFiglia M (1985) The frequency and distribution of medium-sized neurons with indented nuclei in the primate and rodent neostriatum. Brain Res 327:307–311

Hacke W, Zeumer H, Ferbert A, Brückmann H, del Zoppo GJ (1988) Intraarterial thrombolytic therapy improves outcome in patients with acute vertebrobasilar occlusive disease. Stroke 19:1216–1222

Hallenbeck JM (1996) Cellular and molecular mechanisms of ischemic brain damage. In: Siesjo BK, Wieloch T (eds) Inflammatory reactions at the blood-endothelial interface in acute stroke. Lippincott-Raven, Philadelphia, pp 281–300

Hallenbeck JM, Dutka AJ, Tanishima T, Kochanek PM, Kumaroo KK, Thompson CB, Obrenovitch TP, Contreras TJ (1986) Polymorphonuclear leukocyte accumulation in brain regions with low blood flow during the early postischemic period. Stroke 17:246–253

Hamann GF, Okada Y, Fitridge R, del Zoppo GJ (1995) Microvascular basal lamina antigens disappear during cerebral ischemia and reperfusion. Stroke 26:2120–2126

Hamann GF, Okada Y, del Zoppo GJ (1996) Hemorrhagic transformation and microvascular integrity during focal cerebral ischemia/reperfusion. J Cereb Blood Flow Metab 16:1373–1378

Hamann GF, Liebetrau M, Martens H, Burggraf D, Kloss CUA, Bültemeier G, Wunderlich N, Jäger G, Pfefferkorn T (2002) Microvascular basal lamina injury after experimental focal cerebral ischemia and reperfusion in the rat. J Cereb Blood Flow Metab 22:526–533

Haring H-P, Berg EL, Tsurushita N, Tagaya M, del Zoppo GJ (1996) E-selectin appears in nonischemic tissue during experimental focal cerebral ischemia. Stroke 27:1386–1392

Härtl R, Schürer L, Schmid-Schonbein GW, del Zoppo GJ (1996) Experimental antileukocyte interventions in cerebral ischemia. J Cereb Blood Flow Metab 16:1108–1119

Heck LW, Blackburn WD, Irwin MH, Abrahamson DR (1990) Degradation of basement membrane laminin by human neutrophil elastase and cathepsin G. Am J Pathol 136:1267–1274

Heinel L, Rubin S, Rosenwasser R, Vasthare U, Tuma R (1994) Leukocyte involvement in cerebral infarct generation after ischemia and reperfusion. Brain Res Bull 34:137–141

Heo JH, Lucero J, Abumiya T, Koziol JA, Copeland BR, del Zoppo GJ (1999) Matrix metalloproteinases increase very early during experimental focal cerebral ischemia. J Cereb Blood Flow Metab 19:624–633

Hosomi N, Lucero J, Heo JH, Koziol JA, Copeland BR, del Zoppo GJ (2001) Rapid differential endogenous plasminogen activator expression after acute middle cerebral artery occlusion. Stroke 32:1341–1348

ICOS Stroke Trial. ICOS halts trial of stroke drug, reports Q1 net loss. http://biz.yahoo.com/rf/000420/mf.html Accessed 20 April, 2000

Jander S, Schroeter M, Stoll G (2000) Role of NMDA receptor signaling in the regulation of inflammatory gene expression after focal brain ischemia. J Neuroimmunology 109:181–187

Jiang N, Moyle M, Soule H, Rote W, Chopp M (1995) Neutrophil inhibitory factor is neuroprotective after focal ischemia in rats. Ann Neurol 38:935–942

Jiang N, Chopp M, Chahwala S (1998) Neutrophil inhibitory factor treatment of focal cerebral ischemia in the rat. Brain Res 788:25–34

Kawamura S, Schürer L, Goetz A, Kempirski O, Schmucker B, Baethmann A (1990) An improved closed cranial window technique for investigations of blood-brain barrier function and cerebral vasomotor control in the rat. Int J Microcirc Clin Exp 9:369–383

Krane SM (1994) Clinical importance of metalloproteinases and their inhibitors. Ann NY Acad Sci 732:1–10

Kuroiwa T, Ting P, Martinez H, Klatzo I (1985) The aphasic opening of the blood-brain barrier to proteins following temporary middle cerebral artery occlusions. Acta Neuropathol (Berl) 68:122–129

Legos JJ, Whitmore RG, Erhardt JA, Parsons AA, Tuma RF, Barone FC (2000) Quantitative changes in interleukin proteins following focal stroke in the rat. Neuroscience Lett 282:189–192

Lehr H-A, Kress E, Menger M, Friedl H, Hubner C, Arfors K-E (1993) Cigarette smoke elicits leukocytes adhesion to endothelium in hamsters: inhibition by CuZn-SOD. Free Radic Biol Med 14:573–581

Levin EG, del Zoppo GJ (1994) Localization of tissue plasminogen activator in the endothelium of a limited number of vessels. Am J Pathol 144:855–861

Lieberman AP, Pitha PM, Shin HS, Shin ML (1989) Production of tumor necrosis factor and other cytokines by astrocytes stimulated with lipopolysaccharide or a neurotopic virus. Proc Natl Acad Sci USA 86:6348–6352

Little JR, Kerr FWL, Sundt TM Jr (1975) Microcirculatory obstruction in focal cerebral ischemia. Relationship to neuronal alterations. Mayo Clin Proc 50:264–270

Little JR, Kerr FWL, Sundt TM Jr (1976) Microcirculatory obstruction in focal cerebral ischemia: An electron microscopic investigation in monkeys. Stroke 7:25–30

Liu T, Clark RK, McDonnell PC, Young PR, White RF, Barone FC, Feuerstein GZ (1994) Tumor necrosis factor-expression in ischemic neurons. Stroke 25:1481–1488

Liu J, Ginis I, Spatz M, Hallenbeck JM (2000) Hypoxic preconditioning protects cultured neurons against hypoxic stress via TNF-α and ceramide. Am J Physiol Cell Physiol 278:C144–C153

Loddick SA, Wong M-L, Bongiomo PB, Gold PW, Licinio J, Rothwell NJ (1997) Endogenous interleukin-1 receptor antagonist is neuroprotective. Biochem Biophys Res Commun 234:211–215

Matsuo Y, Onodera H, Shiga Y, Nakamura M, Ninomiya M, Kihare T, Kogure K (1994) Correlation between myeloperoxidase-quantified neutrophil accumulation and ischemic brain injury in the rat. Effects of neutrophil depletion. Stroke 25:1469–1475

Meistrell ME, Botchkina GI, Wang H, Di Santo E, Cockroft KM, Bloom O, Vishnubhakat JM, Ghezzi P, Tracey KJ (1997) Tumor necrosis factor is a brain damaging cytokine in cerebral ischemia. Shock 8:341–348

Moossy J (1985) Pathology of ischemic cerebrovascular disease. In: Wilkins RH, Rengachary SS (eds) Neurosurgery/Vol II. McGraw-Hill, New York, pp 1193–1198

Mori E, Tabuchi M, Yoshida T, Yamadori A (1988) Intracarotid urokinase with thromboembolic occlusion of the middle cerebral artery. Stroke 19:802–812

Mori E, Chambers JD, Copeland BR, Arfors K-E, del Zoppo GJ (1992a) Inhibition of polymorphonuclear leukocyte adherence suppresses no-reflow after focal cerebral ischemia. Stroke 23:712–718

Mori E, Yoneda Y, Tabuchi M, Yoshida T, Ohkawa S, Ohsumi Y, Kitano K, Tsutsumi A, Yamadori A (1992b) Intravenous recombinant tissue plasminogen activator in acute carotid artery territory stroke. Neurology 42:976–982

Muchowski P, Zhang L, Chang E, Soule H, Plow E, Moyle M (1994) Functional interaction between the integrin antagonist neutrophil inhibitory factor and the I domain of CD11b/CD18. J Biol Chem 269:26419–26423

Murphy G, Reynolds JJ, Bretz U, Baggiolini M (1987) Collagenase is a component of the specific granules of human neutrophil leukocytes. Biochem J 162:195–197

The National Institutes of Neurological Disorders and Stroke rt-PA Stroke Study Group (1995) Tissue plasminogen activator for acute ischemic stroke. N Engl J Med 333:1581–1587

Nawashiro H, Martin D, Hallenbeck JM (1997a) Neuroprotective effects of TNF-binding protein in focal cerebral ischemia. Brain Res 778:265–271

Nawashiro H, Tasaki K, Ruetzler CA, Hallenbeck JM (1997b) TNF-α pretreatment induces protective effects against focal cerebral ischemia in mice. J Cereb Blood Flow Metab 17:483–490

Ohtsuki T, Ruetzier CA, Tasaki M, Hallenbeck JM (1996) Interleukin-1 mediators induction of tolerance to global ischemia in gerbil hippocampal CA 1 neurones. J Cereb Blood Flow Metab 16:1137–1142

Okada Y, Copeland BR, Fitridge R, Koziol JA, del Zoppo GJ (1994a) Fibrin contributes to microvascular obstructions and parenchymal changes during early focal cerebral ischemia and reperfusion. Stroke 25:1847–1854

Okada Y, Copeland BR, Mori E, Tung M-M, Thomas WS, del Zoppo GJ (1994b) P-selectin and intercellular adhesion molecule-1 expression after focal brain ischemia and reperfusion. Stroke 25:202–211

Okazaki H (1983) Cerebrovascular disease. In: Igaku-Shoin (ed) Fundamentals of neuropathology. New York, pp 25–45

Pike MC, Wicha MS, Yoon P, Mayo L, Boxer LA (1989) Laminin promotes the oxidative burst in human neutrophils via increased chemoattractant receptor expression. J Immunol 142:2004–2011

Pober JS, Cotran RS (1999) Cytokines and endothelial cell biology. Physiol Rev 70:427–451

Ritter L, Orozco J, Coull B, McDonagh P, Rosenblum W (2000) Leukocyte accumulation and hemodynamic changes in the cerebral microcirculation during early reperfusion after stroke. Stroke 31(5):1153–1161

Roberts HR (1992) New perspectives on the coagulation cascade. Hosp Pract 15:97

Rosenberg GA, Navratil M, Barone F, Feuerstein G (1996) Proteolytic cascade enzymes increase in focal cerebral ischemia in rat. J Cereb Blood Flow Metab 16:360–366

Rothwell NJ, Allan S, Toulmond S (1997) The role of interleukin-1 in acute neurodegeneration and stroke: pathophysiological and therapeutic implications. J Clin Invest 100:2648–2652

Ruetzler CA, Furuya K, Takeda H, Hallenbeck JM (2001) Brain vessels normally undergo cyclic activation and inactivation: evidence from tumor necrosis factor-α, heme oxygenase-1, and manganese superoxide dismutase immunostaining of vessels and perivascular brain cells. J Cereb Blood Flow Metab 21:244–252

Saito K, Suyama K, Nishida K, Sei Y, Basile AS (1996) Early increases in TNF-α, IL-6 and IL-1β levels following transient cerebral ischemia in gerbil brain. Neuroscience Lett 206:149–152

Schmid-Schönbein GW (1987a) Capillary plugging by granulocytes and the no-reflow phenomenon in the microcirculation. Fed Proc 46:2397–2401

Schmid-Schönbein GW (1987b) Leukocyte kinetics in the microcirculation. Biorheology 24:139–151

Schmid-Schönbein GW (1990) Leukocyte biophysics. Cell Biophys 17:107–135

Schmid-Schönbein GW, Skalak R, Simon SI, Engler RL (1991) The interaction between leukocytes and endothelium in vivo. Ann N Y Acad Sci 516:348–361

Schneider D, Berrouschot J, Brandt T, Hacke W, Ferbert A, Norris SH, Polmar SH, Schafer E (1998) Safety, pharmocokinetics and biological activity of enlimomab (anti-ICAM-1 antibody): an open-label, dose escalation study in patients hospitalized for acute stroke. Eur Neurol 40(2):78–83

Shohami E, Ginis I, Hallenbeck JM (1999) Dual role of tumor necrosis factor α in brain injury. Cytokine Growth Factor Rev 10:119–130

Soriano SG, Lipton SA, Wang YF, Xiao M, Springer TA, Gutierrez-Ramos J-C, Hickey PR (1996) Intercellular adhesion molecule-1-deficient mice are less susceptible to cerebral ischemia-reperfusion injury. Ann Neurol 39:618–624

Strijbos PJ, Rothwell NJ (1995) Interleukin-1β attenuates excitatory amino acid-induced neurodegeneration in vitro: involvement of nerve growth factor. J Neurosci 15:3468–3474

Tagaya M, Haring H-P, Stuiver I, Wagner S, Abumiya T, Lucero J, Lee P, Copeland BR, Seiffert D, del Zoppo GJ (2001) Rapid loss of microvascular integrin expression during focal brain ischemia reflects neuron injury. J Cereb Blood Flow Metab 21:835–846

Tasaki K, Ruetzler C, Ohtsuki T, Martin D, Nawashiro J, Hallenbeck J (1997) Lipopolysaccharide pretreatment induces resistance against subsequent focal cerebral ischemic damage in spontaneously hypertensive rats. Brain Res 748:267–270

Thomas WS, Mori E, Copeland BR, Yu J-Q, Morrissey JH, del Zoppo GJ (1993) Tissue factor contributes to microvascular defects following cerebral ischemia. Stroke 24:847–853

Todd NV, Picozzi P, Crockard HA, Russell RWR (1986) Duration of ischemia influences the development and resolution of ischemic brain edema. Stroke 17:466–471

Touzani O, Boutin H, Chuquet J, Rothwell N (1999) Potential mechanisms of interleukin-1 involvement in cerebral ischaemia. J Neuroimmunol 100:203–215

Vasthare US, Heinel LA, Rosenwasser RH, Tuma RF (1990) Leukocyte involvement in cerebral ischemia and reperfusion injury. Surg Neurol 33:261–265

von Adrian UK, Chambers JD, McEvoy LM, Bargatze RF, Arfors K-E, Butcher EC (1991) Two-step model of leukocyte-endothelial cell interaction in inflammation: Distinct roles for LECAM-1 and the leukocyte β_2 integrins in vivo. Proc Natl Acad Sci USA 88:7538–7542

Vuorte J, Lindsberg P, Kaste M, Meri S, Jansson S, Rothlein R, Repo H (1999) Anti-ICAM-1 monoclonal antibody R6.5 (Enlimomab) promotes activation of neutrophils in whole blood. J Immunol 162:2353–2357

Walder CE, Green SP, Darbonne WC, Mathias J, Rae J, Dinauer MC, Curnutte JT (1997) Ischemic stroke injury is reduced in mice lacking a functional NADPH oxidate. Stroke 28:2252–2258

Watanabe H, Hattori S, Katsuda S, Nakanishi I, Nagai Y (1990) Human neutrophil elastase: Degradation of basement membrane components and immunolocalization in the tissue. J Biochem 108:753–759

Woodroofe MN, Cuzner ML (1993) Cytokine mRNA expression in inflammatory multiple sclerosis lesions: Detection by nonradioactive in situ hybridization. Cytokine 5:583–588

Yang GY, Gong C, Quin Z, Ye W, Mao Y, Bertz AL (1998) Inhibition of TNF (attenuates infarct volume and ICAM-1 expression in ischemic mouse brain. Neuroreport 9:2131–2134

Yenari M, Kunis D, Sun G, Onley D, Watson L, Turner S, Whitaker S, Steinberg G (1998) Hu23F2G, an antibody recognizing the leukocyte CD11/CD18 integrin, reduces injury in a rabbit model of transient focal cerebral ischemia. Exp Neurol 153:223–233

Yoshida Y, Dereski MO, Garcia JH, Hetzel FW, Chopp M (1992) Photoactivated photofrin II: Astrocytic swelling precedes endothelial injury in rat brain. J Neuropathol Exp Neurol 51:91–100

Zea-Longa E, Weinstein PR, Carlson S, Cummins R (1989) Reversible middle cerebral artery occlusion without craniectomy in rats. Stroke 20:84–91

Zhang R, Chopp M, Zhang Z, Jiang N, Powere C (1998) The expression of P- and E-selectins in three models of middle cerebral artery occlusion. Brain Res 785:207–214

Zhang RL, Chopp M, Li Y, Zaloga C, Jiang N, Jones ML, Miyasaka M, Ward P (1994) Anti-ICAM-1 antibody reduces ischemic cell damage after transient middle cerebral artery occlusion in the rat. Neurology 44:1747–1751

Zhang RL, Chopp M, Jiang N, Tang WX, Prostak J, Manning AM, Anderson DC (1995a) Anti-intercellular adhesion molecule-1 antibody reduces ischemic cell damage after transient but not permanent middle cerebral artery occlusion in the Wistar rat. Stroke 26:1438–1442

Zhang RL, Chopp M, Zaloga C, Zhang ZG, Jiang N, Gautam SC, Tang WX, Tsang W, Anderson DC, Manning AM (1995b) The temporal profiles of ICAM-1 protein and mRNA expression after transient MCA occlusion in the rat. Brain Res 682:182–188

Zhang RL, Chopp M, Zhang ZG, Phillips MC, Rosenbloom CL, Cruz R, Manning A (1996) E-selectin focal cerebral ischemia and reperfusion in the rat. J Cereb Blood Flow Metab 16:1126–1136

Zülch K-J, Kleihues P (1966) Neuropathology of cerebral infarction. Stroke. Thule International Symposia 1966. Nordiska Bokhandelns, Stockholm, pp 57–75

10 Inflammation-Mediated Damage as a Potential Therapeutic Target in Acute Ischemic Stroke

Á. Chamorro, A.M. Planas

10.1 Introduction

Stroke represents worldwide one of the leading medical problems but the acute treatment of this condition remains challenging as no single drug has unequivocally demonstrated to be effective (Adams et al. 1994; The European Ad Hoc Consensus Group 1996). Intravenous thrombolysis with rt-PA is the only FDA-approved therapy for stroke during the first 3 h after clinical onset. Recently, European health authorities have also approved its use in the European Union for stroke patients with symptoms lasting no more than 3 h. However, as the majority of stroke patients receive neurological attention at a longer than 3 h delay from symptom onset, the epidemiological impact of thrombolysis is at this stage only marginal.

The earliest events that follow the onset of ischemia would be the accumulation of Na^+/Ca^{2+} ions consequent to loss of membrane potential and unregulated ion fluxes, massive release of excitotoxic neurotransmitters, and oxidative stress that leads to radical formation, lipid peroxidation, and membrane and organelle damage (Feuerstein and Wang 2001). Given the protracted delay that stroke patients sustain before they receive initial medical attention, it can be presumed that these events are already in place in most instances. Besides, if the intensity and/or the duration of ischemia is maintained, these events are shortly followed by processes such as de novo gene expression, activation of microglia, and infiltration of blood borne leukocytes across the blood brain barrier into the brain (Del Zoppo et al. 2001). The underlying basic mechanisms that lead to clinical worsening during the acute phase of stroke are not well understood. Early progression of neurological symptoms occurs in 25%–40% of ischemic stroke patients in prospective studies and is associated with increased mortality and permanent functional disability (Dávalos et al. 1990; Toni et al. 1995; Jorgensen et al. 1994). Clinical, radiological, and biochemical factors have been described as potential predictors of early neurological deterioration but with a limited predicted value. Some cellular reactions contribute to expand neuronal injury, including excitatory amino acids release, iron accumulation, oxygen free radicals and nitric oxide production, or apoptosis (Castillo 1999). During the last few years, a body of evidence has also stressed the role of inflammation in the pathophysiology of acute brain ischemia, although many questions remain concerning the relevance of neuroinflammation in human stroke (DeGraba 1998). It is the main aim of this article to review whether the well-established participation of inflammatory damage in experimental stroke corresponds well with the events that take place at the bedside. In addition, this article analyzes if the participation of these inflammatory changes varied across the main stroke subtypes that are encountered in the clinic.

10.2 Differences Between Stroke Patients and Experimental Models of Ischemic Stroke

A note a caution is necessary when estimating whether the findings observed in experimental models of brain ischemia are also observed in the clinic. In the former setting, most variables can be strictly controlled and monitored; in the latter, patients are frequently surrounded by a significant amount of biological uncertainty or unmeasured effects. Factors often disregarded in the lab but of great concern in the clinic are the prevalence of environmental factors, such older age, gender, diabetes, hypertension, or dyslipemia, among others. Stroke patients may be exposed to identifiable risk factors that can be adjusted for in multivariate predictor models of functional outcome. However, the duration or intensity of exposure to these factors is frequently impossible to measure. Moreover, patients could be influenced by genes that sway not only the risk of stroke but also the traits of the hemodynamic response, the strength of thrombotic or antithrombotic factors, the inflammatory prowess, or the antioxidant capacity. To further entangle the state of affairs, stroke may result in the clinic from a large list of causes and mechanisms, and in as many as 30%–40% of instances the cause of symptoms remains unraveled despite a comprehensive diagnostic workup. Identical stroke subtypes may nevertheless bring about dissimilar consequences in otherwise comparable patients, as vessels of variable caliber may become occluded for varied lengths of time. Patients may harbor emboli of protean thrombogenicity and susceptibility to lysis and this can also translate into larger or smaller infarctions. These elements must be kept in mind to understand why so many encouraging observations obtained experimentally were followed by frustrating results in the clinic.

No more trivial for an accurate understanding of the frustrating results of clinical trials in acute ischemic stroke are the proper limitations of the neurologic examination. Unlike the relatively objective measurement of brain infarction volumes in animals, the tool that determines the clinical fate of patients relies on a neurological examination whose reliability may be jeopardized by several caveats. Patients with infarctions located in certain strategic areas, such as the medial frontal lobe, the inferior parietal lobe, or the thalamus, may manifest severe deficits which clinicians might misinterpret as paralysis when they really attest motor neglect secondary to disruption of motor planning areas in the brain (Chamorro et al. 1997). To elucidate the neurobiological nature of motor impairment is important because motor neglect tends to be short-lived without therapeutic interventions, whereas the paralysis is more reluctant to spontaneous recovery. If patients with neglect or paralysis are not well balanced in a stroke trial the actual value of an experimental therapy could be misled by a wrong clinical assessment. Another limitation of the clinical exam is the ceiling effect of neurological worsening, implying an easier detection of clinical worsening in patients with milder impairments at the start of treatment. Although the motor score of a hemiplegic patient cannot worsen further as a result of ceiling, clinical stability does not preclude "molecular worsening" within the penumbra and this could affect the extent of cellular recovery.

10.3 Inflammation as a Therapeutic Target for Stroke Patients

Most of the inflammatory reactions are mediated by cytokines, small glycoproteins expressed by many cell types in response to acute cerebral ischemia. Cytokines play an important role in several inflammatory reactions, resulting in adhesion molecule upregulation, recruitment and activation of leukocytes, promotion of leukocyte-endothelium interaction and conversion of the local endothelium to a prothrombotic state. Increases of proinflammatory cytokines (IL-1β, TNF-a, and IL-6) have been detected in the ischemic cortex 1 h after middle cerebral artery (MCA) occlusion in experimental models of brain ischemia (Yamasaki et al. 1995). Intraventricular injection of IL-1β and TNF-a in rats enlarges infarct size and brain edema after MCA occlusion, whereas the injection of antibodies against IL-1β and TNF-a reduces injury (Barone et al. 1997). In stroke patients, several studies have reported elevations of proinflammatory cytokines in peripheral blood (Beamer et al. 1995; Fassbender et al. 1994; Vila et al. 1999; Tarkowski et al. 1995; Kim et al. 1996; Farrarese et al. 1999), as well in cerebrospinal fluid (CSF; Tarkowski et al. 1997).

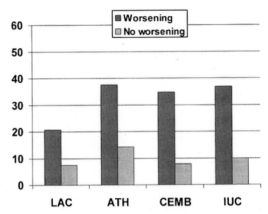

Fig. 1. IL-6 in plasma in patients with all stroke subtypes. *LAC*, lacunar infarct (*n* = 33); *ATH*, atherosclerotic infarct (*n* = 84); *CEMB*, cardioembolic infarct (*n* = 76); *IUC*, infarct of undetermined cause (*n* = 38)

We evaluated whether proinflammatory cytokines lead to early progression of neurological symptoms in patients with acute ischemic stroke (Vila et al. 2000). The study population included 231 patients consecutively admitted with first-ever ischemic cerebral infarction within the first 24 h from onset. Neurological worsening was defined when the Canadian Stroke Scale (CSS) score fell at least 1 point during the first 48 h after admission (Chamorro et al. 1995). IL-6 and TNF-*a* were determined in plasma and cerebrospinal fluid (CSF; *n* = 81) obtained on admission. Eighty-three patients (35.9%) deteriorated within the first 48 h. Using multiple logistic regression we found that IL-6 in plasma (> 21.5 pg/ml; OR 37.7, CI 11.9 to 118.8) or in CSF (> 6.3 pg/ml; OR 13.1, CI 2.2 to 77.3) were independent factors for early clinical worsening. The association was statistically significant in all ischemic stroke subtypes (Fig. 1) as well as in subjects with cortical or subcortical infarctions (Fig. 2). IL-6 in plasma was highly correlated with body temperature, glucose, fibrinogen, and infarct volume. In addition, CSF and plasma concentrations of TNF-*a* were also higher in patients who deteriorated, but the differences observed did not remain significant on multivariate analysis. As shown in Table 1, we had previously dem-

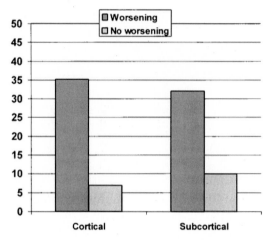

Fig. 2. Patients with clinical deterioration had significantly increased levels of IL-6 in plasma compared with patients without clinical deterioration in cortical ($n=77$, $p<0.01$) and subcortical ($n=99$, $p<0.01$) infarcts

Table 1. Independent predictors of stroke outcome including and excluding lesion size on CT scan

Variable	CT scan				No CT scan			
	β	SE	p	r	β	SE	p	r
Volume	1.5	0.55	.0001	.15	. . .	. . .	. . .	. . .
Mathew score	4.05	1.05	.0001	.23	4.56	1.04	.000	.26
Improvement	1.42	0.53	.007	.15	1.61	0.46	.000	.20
ESR	1.08	0.52	.04	.09	1.23	0.47	.009	.13

ESR, erythrocyte sedimentation rate.

onstrated that the erythrocyte sedimentation rate (ESR), a measure of the intensity of the acute-phase response started by IL-6, was an independent predictor of poor clinical outcome independent of infarct size and clinical severity on admission. Based on these findings we may conclude that in addition to participation in the acute-phase response that follows focal cerebral ischemia, an increased level of

IL-6 at hospital entry equally reflects the extent of tissue damage and the risk of further tissue disruption and clinical worsening. Further, this relationship is applicable to patients with any of the most frequent stroke subtypes without regard to the initial size or topography of the ischemic infarction.

10.4 The Special Case of Lacunar Stroke

Lacunar stroke represents a well-defined stroke subtype diagnosed in 25–30% of all strokes. They consist of small, deep cavities caused by microatheroma, lipohyalinosis, or fibrinoid necrosis in small penetrating branches of large cerebral arteries, initially described in chronic hypertensive individuals (Chamorro et al. 1991). While accumulating evidence suggests that inflammatory-mediated damage plays a role in brain ischemia, it remains unclear whether inflammation also intervenes in lacunar stroke progression and outcome. In 113 consecutive patients with a lacunar infarction documented by CT scan or brain MRI, we assessed biochemical factors of early neurological deterioration (Castellanos et al. 2002). IL-6, TNF-α, and ICAM-1 were determined by ELISA in blood samples obtained on admission. Cytokine determinations were performed blinded to clinical and radiological data. Plasma glutamate and GABA levels were also quantified by high-performance liquid chromatography. Because cytokine levels were not normally distributed, the Spearman correlation coefficient was used to analyze the association between cytokines and temperature, fibrinogen, glucose, and infarct volume. Cutoff values for IL-6 with the highest sensitivity and specificity in plasma and CSF were calculated as described by Roberts et al. (Robert et al. 1991), given the different distribution of IL-6 according to outcome groups. All three inflammatory molecules were significantly increased in patients compared with controls, as shown in Table 2. Similar levels of proinflammatory molecules were found between groups classified by the suspected cause of lacunar stroke, lacunar syndrome, and the presence or not of the main stroke risk factors, such as hypertension, diabetes mellitus, atrial fibrillation, prior stroke, or transient ischemic attack (data not shown). Significant correlations were found between glutamate and GABA levels and the

Table 2. Median [quartiles] concentrations of inflammatory markers in patients with lacunar infarctions and control subjects

	Patients ($n=113$)	Controls ($n=43$)	p Value
IL-6, pg/ml	13.9 [9.2,23.8]	3.1 (1.3,4.1)	<0.001
TNF-a, pg/ml	8.2 [6.4,15.3]	7.0 (5.7,8.4)	0.001
ICAM-1, pg/ml	167 [140,207]	187 (172,223)	0.015

Table 3. Odds ratio of early neurological deterioration for inflammatory markers after adjustment for serum glutamate and GABA concentrations

Odds ratio (95% CI)

Variables	Model A	Model B	Model C
TNF-a>14 pg/ml	39 (4.6–336)	28 (3.0–266)	37 (1.6–863)
ICAM-1>208 pg/ml	125 (14.7–1,067)	76 (8.1–712)	70 (3.0–1,594)
Glutamate >200 μmol/l	*****	11 (2.1–59)	*****
GABA<240 nmol/l	*****	*****	184 (11.7–2,893)

Model A was not adjusted for neurotransmitters; model B was adjusted for serum glutamate concentrations; model C for serum GABA concentrations. Cutoff values were calculated by the method of Robert et al. (see Methods).

concentrations of IL-6 ($r=0.46$ and $r=-0.47$), TNF-a ($r=0.39$ and $r=-0.42$) and ICAM-1 ($r=0.34$ and $r=-0.44$) (all p values <0.001). Early neurological deterioration was recorded in 27 patients (23.9%) and poor outcome in 26 (23%). Median (quartiles) concentrations in plasma of TNF-a, IL-6, and ICAM-1 were significantly higher in patients who had early neurological deterioration than in those with nonprogressing strokes ($p<0.001$), as shown in Fig. 3. Significant differences were also observed between patients with poor and good outcome at 3 months (Fig. 3). Logistic regression analysis after adjusting for potential confounders showed that TNF-a >14 pg/ml and ICAM-1>208 pg/ml were independently associated both with early neurological deterioration (OR, 511; 95% CI, 17–4,937; $p<0.001$ and OR, 315; 95% CI, 17–5,748; $p<0.001$, respectively) and poor outcome at 3 months (OR, 3.0; 95% CI, 1.0–8.5; $p=0.042$ and OR, 4.2; 95% CI, 1.3–13.6; $p<0.015$, respectively). Therefore, higher

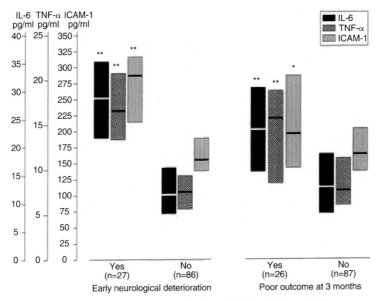

Fig. 3. Median values and quartiles (25% and 75%) of plasma inflammatory markers by early clinical course and outcome at 3 months. *$p<0.05$; **$p<0.001$

concentrations of TNF-a and ICAM-1 in blood were associated with early neurological deterioration and poor functional outcome in lacunar infarctions, suggesting that inflammation also contributes to brain injury in lacunar stroke. As previous studies had also found a relationship between neurotransmitter amino acids and the progression of lacunar infarctions (Serena et al. 2001), the odds of early neurological deterioration for TNF-a and ICAM-1 were further adjusted for plasma glutamate and GABA concentrations. However, the odds ratios of early neurological deterioration for TNF-a and ICAM-1 did not change after adjustment for plasma glutamate and GABA concentrations, as shown in Table 3.

10.5 Genetic Susceptibility to Inflammatory Damage

The likely implication of genetic susceptibility to inflammatory damage was recently suggested by our group in a case control study of
patients with lacunar stroke (Revilla et al. 2002). In particular, we
analyzed the contribution of a base pair substitution $-174G/C$ in the
promoter region of the IL-6 gene that regulates IL-6 gene expression. The $-174G/C$ polymorphism of the IL-6 gene is thought to be
a functional polymorphism that determines differences in the degree
of IL-6 gene expression to stressful stimuli between individuals. The
C allele has been associated with significantly lower plasma levels
of IL-6 and lower IL-6 gene expression, maybe because the C allele
at position -174 creates a binding site for the transcription factor
NF-1 that acts as a repressor of gene expression. We compared the
prevalence of this polymorphism in 83 patients with lacunar stroke
and in an age- and sex-matched cohort of asymptomatic controls.
The prevalence of CC genotype (18.3% vs. 7.3%, $p=0.03$), and the
frequency of C allele (42.7% vs. 31.1%, $p=0.03$) were statistically
significantly higher in patients with lacunar stroke than in asymptomatic controls. A logistic regression model showed that independent
variables associated with lacunar stroke included history of hypertension, diabetes, hyperlipidemia, smoking, and CC genotype of the
$-174G/C$ IL-6 gene polymorphism (OR, 4.28). Pending validation in
a larger population, these results suggest a genetic susceptibility to
inflammatory damage in lacunar infarction in concert with atherosclerotic risk factors.

10.6 The Role of Anti-inflammation in Acute Stroke

IL-10 is an anti-inflammatory molecule, mainly secreted by lymphocytes and monocytes/macrophages, that blocks proinflammatory actions (Tedgui and Mallat 2001). IL-10 inhibits leukocyte adhesion to
IL-1 activated human endothelial cells, an effect that correlated with
a decrease in endothelial ICAM-1 and VCAM-1 expression. IL-10
also suppresses the production of IL-1, IL-6, IL-8, and TNF-a. In
monocytes, IL-10 selectively inhibits NF-κB activation (Malefyt et

Table 4. Levels of interleukin-10 according to infarct topography and stroke subtypes

	Number	IL-10		p Value
Infarct topography				NS
Cortical	77	6.1	(2.1)	
Subcortical	99	5.9	(2.3)	
Stroke subtypes				NS
Cardioembolic	76	5.9	(1.9)	
Lacunar	33	6.2	(2.5)	
Atherosclerotic	84	5.7	(2.2)	
Undetermined	38	6.3	(2.2)	

IL-10 levels are expressed as mean (SD) in pg/ml.

al. 1991). IL-10-deficient mice have an increased stroke lesion size after occlusion of the middle cerebral artery (Grilli et al. 2000), whereas rats treated with IL-10 have a decreased stroke lesion size (Spera et al. 1998). In patients with acute stroke, a transient increase in IL-10 concentrations in plasma, CSF, and blood mononuclear cells have been detected (Tarkowski et al. 1997). However, it was unclear whether IL-10 levels were associated with the risk of early stroke progression. We collected blood samples of 231 patients with acute stroke admitted within 24 h from stroke onset for IL-10 determinations with a commercially available quantitative immunoassay (quantikine; Vila et al. 2003). Samples were collected within 6 h from symptom onset in 50% of cases and within 12 h in 80% of cases. Eighty-three patients (35.9%) worsened within the first 48 h after stroke onset. No differences in IL-10 were observed according to stroke subtype or topography, as shown in Table 4. Contrarily, significantly lower concentrations of IL-10 were found in patients with neurological worsening ($p < 0.05$). Lower plasma concentrations of IL-10 (<6 pg/mL) were associated with clinical worsening on multivariate analysis (odds ratio = 3.1, 95% CI = 1.1–8.9) independently of hyperthermia, hyperglycemia, or neurological condition on admission, as shown in Table 5. Further analysis disclosed that early worsening was independently associated with lower IL-10 plasma levels in patients with subcortical infarcts or lacunar stroke but not in patients with cortical lesions (Figs. 4, 5). Thus, if these findings are

Table 5. Factors associated to neurological deterioration

Variable	β	SE	OR	(95% CI)
IL-10<6 pg/ml	1.17	0.52	3.2	(1.1–8.9)
Body temperature (°C)	3.39	0.59	29.9	(9.5–94.6)
Canadian Stroke Score	0.44	0.13	1.5	(1.2–2.0)
Serum glucose (mg/dl)	0.02	0.005	1.02	(1.01–1.03)

Other variables included in the model were: age, sex, total leukocyte count, admission delay, and presence of early infarct signs on brain CT scan.

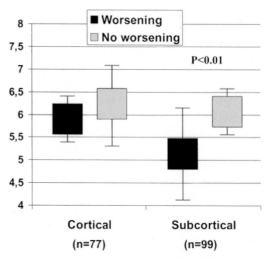

Fig. 4. IL-10 plasma levels (pg/ml) and neurological worsening according to stroke topography. Patients with neurological worsening had significantly reduced levels of IL-10 in plasma compared with patients without neurological worsening only in subcortical infarcts ($n=99$; $p<0.01$) but not in cortical infarcts ($n=77$)

validated, patients with lacunar infarcts would represent ideal candidates to participate in clinical trials of neuroprotection using anti-inflammatory drugs.

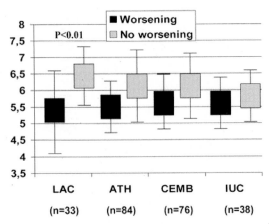

Fig. 5. IL-10 plasma levels (pg/ml) and neurological worsening according to stroke etiology. *LAC* indicates lacunar infarct ($n=33$); *ATH*, atherosclerotic infarct ($n=84$); *CEMB*, cardioembolic infarct ($n=76$); *IUC*, infarct of undetermined cause ($n=38$)

10.7 Understanding Heparin as an Anti-inflammatory Agent in Acute Ischemic Stroke

The evidence favoring or discouraging the administration of adjusted-dose UFH to patients with ischemic stroke is scanty (Cerebral Embolism Study Group 1983; Duke et al. 1986; Dobkin 1983). Available data on "immediate" anticoagulation is also inadequate. Clashing with the widespread opinion of the limited value of UFH (Chamorro et al. 1995) in acute ischemic stroke, a few studies emphasized the relevance of dose-adjusted UFH, and treatment expeditiousness (Chamorro et al. 1999). Thus, recovery was greater in patients treated within 6 h from symptoms onset, and stroke recurrence and serious bleeding were associated to abnormal coagulation tests. We also showed a lower total leukocyte count in patients anticoagulated with UFH than in those receiving aspirin (Chamorro et al. 2000).

In murine brain ischemia, higher anticoagulant doses (Yanaka et al. 1996a), and shorter anticoagulation delays (Yanaka et al. 1996b) are necessary to reduce infarction volume. We believe that these

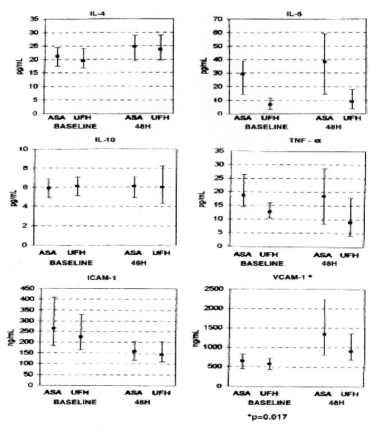

Fig. 6. Longitudinal time course of inflammatory concentration levels (medians and quartiles) in patients with ischemic stroke treated with UFH or aspirin

conditions are also essential to isolate the anti-inflammatory properties of UFH in man (Chamorro 2001).

Aiming to achieve this goal, we evaluated the anti-inflammatory effects of UFH and aspirin in 167 patients with acute ischemic stroke (Chamorro et al. 2002). Blood samples were collected before the onset of antithrombotic therapy (less than 24 h from symptom onset), and after 48 h by personnel unaware of the clinical and thera-

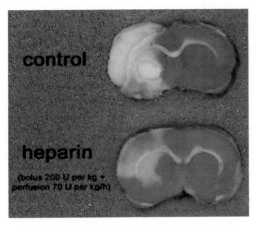

Fig. 7. Marked reduction of infarction volume in the rat brain after the administration of unfractionated heparin

peutic data. IL-6, IL-10, IL-4, TNF-a, soluble ICAM-1 (sICAM-1), and soluble VCAM-1 (sVCAM-1) concentrations in plasma were measured in the same laboratory with commercially available quantitative sandwich enzyme-linked immunoadsorbent assays (Quantikine, R&D System, Minneapolis, MN). Outcome was evaluated using stepwise logistic regression analyses. After adjusting for baseline inflammatory values, baseline neurological score, baseline CT scan, and mean arterial pressure, values of sVCAM-1 were on average 1.24 (95% CI, 1.04–1.49; $p=0.017$) higher in the aspirin group than in the heparin group. The time course of the remaining biological parameters did not differ between the two antithrombotic groups, as depicted in Fig. 6. Regardless of the initial severity of neurological symptoms and admission CT findings, we found an inverse relationship between increased sVCAM-1 at follow-up and the chances of full functional recovery. Namely, a twofold increment of baseline sVCAM-1 levels at 48 h doubled the odds of poor outcome.

VCAM-1 is an adhesion factor intensely expressed by human astrocytes and endothelial cells from infarcted tissue (Blann et al. 1999) that induces tissue factor (TF) expression (McGilvray et al. 1997). Following the release of cytokines, TF is the primary cellular initiator of the coagulation cascade in vivo and represents a hemostatic envelope diffusely expressed in human cortex and cerebral vessels (Drake et al. 1989). VCAM-1 is also expressed following endothelial activation by cytokines that selectively bind mononuclear cells such as lymphocytes and monocytes (Von Andrian 2001).

As shown in Fig. 7, we found smaller infarction volumes in focal ischemic rats treated with UHF than in controls whenever treatment was provided within 3 h from transient middle cerebral artery occlusion. The agent was given at doses equivalent to those administered to patients (0.3–0.6 U/ml; pending publication). Investigations currently performed at our lab also suggest that volume reduction in the rat brain is significantly associated with a decrease in VCAM-1 (data not shown).

10.8 Conclusions

We provide data reinforcing the clinical relevance of neuroinflammation in human ischemic stroke. Our results indicate that the levels of IL-6 in plasma or in CSF are independent factors for early stroke worsening. CSF and plasma concentrations of TNF-α are also higher in stroke patients who deteriorate, but the differences observed do not remain significant when multivariate analysis is performed to control for the effect of confounders. Nevertheless, in patients with lacunar stroke, higher concentrations of TNF-α and ICAM-1 in blood are associated with early neurological deterioration and poor functional outcome at 3 months. Besides, it seems plausible that genetic susceptibility to inflammatory damage, in concert with atherosclerotic risk factors, plays a role in the genesis of lacunar infarction. Although no differences in baseline IL-10 are observed among patients according to the subtype or topography of the stroke, significantly lower concentrations of IL-10 are found in patients with neurological worsening. The inverse association is particularly prominent in patients with lacunar infarction or subcortical strokes. Based on these data, it can be concluded that therapeutic interventions aimed at modulating inflammatory processes after ischemic stroke are justified. Our findings would support interventions aimed at decreasing IL-6 (all ischemic strokes), TNF-α and ICAM-1 (lacunar stroke), VCAM-1 (nonlacunar stroke). Interventions directed at increasing IL-10 might be useful in patients with subcortical stroke or lacunar infarctions. At last, UFH stands as one of the interventions that deserves appropriate testing in the clinic.

Acknowledgements. This work is indebted to a long list of colleagues but we want to emphasize the contribution of Drs J. Castillo, A. Dávalos, N. Vila, A. Cervera, JC Reverter, and C. Justicia. Grants 00/0640 and 01/1150 from the Fondo de Investigaciones Sanitarias of the Spanish Ministry of Health are also acknowledged.

References

Adams HP, Brott TG, Crowell RM, Furlan AJ, Gomez CR, Grotta J, Helgason CM, Marler JR, Woolson RF, Zivin JA, Feinberg W, Mayberg M (1994) Guidelines for the management of patients with acute ischemic stroke. A statement for healthcare professionals from a special writing group of the Stroke Council, American Heart Association. Stroke 25:1901–1914

Barone FC, Arvin B, White RF, Miller A, Webb CL, Willette RN, Lysko PG, Feuerstein GZ (1997) Tumor necrosis factor-a. A mediator of focal ischemic brain injury. Stroke 28:1233–1244

Beamer NB, Coull BM, Clark WM, Hazel JS, Silberger JR (1995) Interleukin-6 and interleukin-1 receptor antagonist in acute stroke. Ann Neurol 37:800–804

Blann A, Kumar P, Krupinski J, McCollum C, Beevers DG, Lip GY (1999) Soluble intercellular adhesion molecule-1, E-selectin, vascular cell adhesion molecule-1 and von Willebrand factor in stroke. Blood Coagul Fibrinolysis 10:277–284

Castellanos M, Castillo J, García MM, Leira R, Serena J, Chamorro A, Dávalos A (2002) Inflammation-mediated damage in progressing lacunar infarctions. A potential therapeutic target. Stroke 33:982–987

Castillo J (1999) Deteriorating stroke: diagnostic criteria, predictors, mechanisms and treatment. Cerebrovasc Dis 9:1–8

Cerebral Embolism Study Group (1983) Immediate anticoagulation and embolic stroke. A randomized trial. Stroke 14:668–676

Chamorro A (2001) Immediate anticoagulation in acute focal brain ischemia revisited: gathering the evidence. Stroke 32:577–578

Chamorro A, Sacco RL, Mohr JP, Foulkes MA, Kase CS, Tatemichi TK, Wolf PA, Price TR, Hier DB (1991) Lacunar infarction: Clinical-CT correlations in the Stroke Data Bank. Stroke 22:175–181

Chamorro A, Vila N, Saiz A, Alday M, Tolosa E (1995) Early anticoagulation after large cerebral infarction: a safety study. Neurology 45:861–865

Chamorro A; Vila N; Ascaso C; Saiz A; Alonso P; Montalvo J; Tolosa E (1995) Early prediction of stroke severity: Role of the erythrocyte sedimentation rate. Stroke 26:573–576

Chamorro A, Marshall RS, Valls-Sole J, Tolosa E, Mohr JP (1997) Motor behavior in stroke patients with isolated medial frontal ischemic infarction. Stroke 28:1755–1760

Chamorro A, Vila N, Ascaso C, Blanc R (1999) Heparin in acute stroke with atrial fibrillation. Clinical relevance of very early treatment. Arch Neurol 56:1098–1102

Chamorro A, Obach V, Vila N, Revilla M, Cervera A, Ascaso C (2000) A comparison of the acute-phase response in patients with ischemic stroke treated with high-dose heparin or aspirin. J Neurol Sci 178:17–22

Chamorro A, Cervera A, Castillo J, Dávalos A, Aponte JJ, Planas AM (2002) Unfractionated heparin is associated with a lower rise of serum vascular cell adhesion molecule-1 in acute ischemic stroke patients. Neurosci Lett 328:229–232

Dávalos A, Cendra E, Teruel J, Martinez M, Genis D (1990) Deteriorating ischemic stroke: risk factors and prognosis. Neurology 40:1865–1869

DeGraba TJ (1998) The role of inflammation after acute stroke. Neurology 51:S62–S68

Del Zoppo GJ, Hecker KJ, Hallenbeck JM (2001) Inflammation after stroke: is it harmful? Arch Neurol 58:669–672

Dobkin BH (1983) Heparin for lacunar stroke in progression. Stroke 14:421–423

Drake TA, Morrissey JH, Edgington TS (1989) Selective cellular expression of tissue factor in human tissues. Implications for disorders of homeostasis and thrombosis. Am J Pathol 134:1087–1097

Duke RJ, Bloch RF, Turpie AG, Trebilcock R, Bayer N (1986) Intravenous heparin for the prevention of stroke progression in acute partial stable stroke. Ann Intern Med 105:825–828

The European Ad Hoc Consensus Group (1996) European strategies for early intervention in stroke. Cerebrovasc Dis 6:315–324

Farrarese C, Mascarucci P, Zoia C, Cavarretta R, Frigoo M, Begni B, Sarinella F, Frattola L, De Simoni MG (1999) Increased cytokine release from peripheral blood cells after acute stroke. J Cereb Blood Flow Metab 19:1004–1009

Fassbender K, Rossol S, Kammer T, Daffertshofer M, Wirth S, Dollman M, Hennerici M (1994) Proinflammatory cytokines in serum of patients with acute cerebral ischemia: kinetics of secretion and relation to the extent of brain damage and outcome of disease. J Neurol Sci 122:135–139

Feuerstein GZ, Wang X (2001) New opportunities for stroke prevention and therapeutics: a hope from anti-inflammatory drugs? In: Feuerstein GZ (ed) Inflammation and stroke. Birkhäuser Verlag Basel, pp 3–10

Grilli M., Barbieri I, Basudev H, Brusa R, Casati C, Lozza G, Ongini E (2000) Interleukin-10 modulates neuronal threshold of vulnerability to ischemic damage. Eur J Neurosci 12:2265–2272

Jorgensen HS, Nakayama H, Raaschou HO, Olsen TS (1994) Effect of blood pressure and diabetes on stroke in progression. Lancet 344:156–159

Kim JS, Yoon SS, Kim YH, Ryu JS (1996) Serial measurement of interleukin-6, transforming growth factor-β and S-100 protein in patients with acute stroke. Stroke 27:1553–1557

Malefyt RW, Abrams J, Bennet B, Figdor CG, Vries JE (1991) Interleukin-10 inhibits cytokine synthesis by human monocytes. J Exp Med 174:1209–1220

McGilvray ID, Lu Z, Bitar R, Dackiw APB, Davreux CJ, Rotsein OD (1997) VLA-4 integrin cross-linking on human monocytic THP-1 cells induces tissue factor expression by a mechanism involving mitogen-activated protein kinase. J Biol Chem 272:10287–10294

Revilla M, Obach V, Cervera A, Dávalos A, Castillo J, Chamorro A (2002) A-174G/C polymorphism of the interleukin-6 gene in patients with lacunar infarction. Neurosc Lett 324:29–32

Robert C, Vermont J, Bosson JL (1991) Formulas for threshold computations. Comput Biomed Res 24:514–519

Serena J, Leira R, Castillo J, Pumar JM, Castellanos M, Dávalos A (2001) Neurological deterioration in acute lacunar infarctions: the role of excitatory and inhibitory neurotransmitters. Stroke 32:1154–1161

Spera PA, Ellison JA, Feuerstein GZ, Barone FC (1998) IL-10 reduces rat brain injury following focal stroke. Neurosci Lett 251:189–192

Tarkowski E, Rosengren L, Blomstrand C, Wikkelsö C, Jensen C, Ekholm S, Tarkowski A (1995) Early intrathecal production of interleukin-6 predicts the size of brain lesion in stroke. Stroke 26:1393–1398

Tarkowski E, Rosengren L, Blomstrand C, Wikkelsö C, Jensen C, Tarkowski E, Rosengren L, Blomstrand C, Wikkelsö C, Jensen C, Ekholm S, Tarkowski A (1997) Intrathecal release of pro- and anti-inflammatory cytokines during stroke. Clin Exp Immunol 110:492–499

Tedgui A, Mallat Z (2001) Anti-inflammatory mechanisms in the vascular wall. Circ Res 88:877–887

Toni D, Fiorelli M, Gentile M, Bastianello S, Sacchetti ML, Argentino C, Pozzilli C, Fischi C (1995) Progressing neurological deficit secondary to acute ischemic stroke: a study on predictability, pathogenesis, and prognosis. Arch Neurol 52:670–675

Vila N, Filella X, Deulofeu R, Ascaso C, Abellana R, Chamorro A (1999) Cytokine-induced inflammation and long-term stroke functional outcome. J Neurol Sci 162:185–188

Vila N, Castillo J, Dávalos A, Chamorro A (2000) Proinflammatory cytokines and early neurological worsening in ischemic stroke. Stroke 31:2325–2329

Vila N, Castillo J, Dávalos A, Esteve A, Planas A, Chamorro A (2003) Levels of anti-inflammatory cytokines and neurological worsening in acute ischemic stroke. Stroke 34:671–675

Von Andrian UH (2001) The immunoglobulin superfamily in leukocyte recruitment. In: Collins T (ed) Leukocyte recruitment, endothelial cell adhesion molecules, and transcriptional control. Insights for drug discovery. Kluwer Academic Publishers, Norwell, MA, pp 55–107

Yamasaki Y, Matsuura N, Shozuhara H, Onodera H, Itoyama Y, Kogure K (1995) Interleukin-1 as a pathogenic mediator of ischemic brain damage in rats. Stroke 26:676–681

Yanaka K, Spellman R, McCarthy JB, Low WC, Camarata PJ (1996a) Reduction of brain injury using heparin to inhibit leukocyte accumulation in a rat model of transient focal cerebral ischemia. II. Dose-response effect and the therapeutic window. J Neurosurg 85:1108–1112

Yanaka K, Spellman SR, McCarthy JB, Oegema TR, Low WC, Camarata PJ (1996b) Reduction of brain injury using heparin to inhibit leukocyte accumulation in a rat model of transient focal cerebral ischemia. I. Protective mechanism. J Neurosurg 85:1102–1107

11 Design Issues in Selected Recent or Ongoing Stroke Trials

M. Schwaninger, P. Ringleb, W. Hacke

11.1 Introduction

The basic science of cerebral ischemia is complex and involves multiple systems. As reviewed elsewhere, hypoperfusion, excitotoxicity, inflammation, and apoptosis are the main disease mechanisms that are tackled by pharmacological interventions. A large number of agents and strategies has been developed to change the pathophysiological cascade. While it has been a rather easy task to find agents that would work in the experimental setting, translation into the clinic has been a major problem. After more than two decades of dedicated clinical trials, only a single agent, rt-PA, has been approved by national agencies for routine use. This review will discuss pitfalls of prior clinical trials and the promise of upcoming strategies in clinical testing.

11.2 Choice of Agent

So far, all the clinical studies that have had a positive result were concerned with vascular aspects of stroke (Kay et al. 1995; Ninds Rt-Pa Stroke Study Group 1995; Furlan et al. 1999; Sherman et al. 2000). All neuroprotective agents have failed in the clinic so far, although there are lots of agents available that reduce the infarct size in experimental animal models of focal cerebral ischemia. For the selection of neuroprotective agents it seems to hold true: the wider the choice, the greater the trouble. In this situation, early studies have made obvious mistakes in the choice of agents. Antiexcitotoxic agents are effective in experimental models but have a small therapeutic ratio (the ratio of doses producing therapeutic effects and side effects; Dawson et al. 2001). This resulted in the administration of subefficacious doses in order to avoid the emergence of side effects. For future trials, compounds with a sufficient therapeutic ratio well above 1 have to be selected. However, it is often difficult to foresee potential side effects in the preclinic phase. Also, the dose–response relationship of effects and side effects depends on the species. Therefore, only the early clinical phases will clarify whether effective doses are tolerated by humans. Recent stroke studies paid special attention to the dose–response relationship. For the ongoing Repinotan trial, a bedside test device was specifically developed to determine drug concentrations. The DIAS trial followed a dose-ranging design investigating three fixed doses (25 mg, 37.5 mg, and 50 mg) in parallel. An interim analysis, however, showed an unacceptable rate of intracerebral hemorrhage with doses of 25 mg or higher. Consequently, a dose escalation design has been adopted starting with a dose of 62.5 microgram/kg body weight. The AbBEST trial was a phase IIb trial that based the dose selection on a phase IIa dose finding trial (The Abciximab in Ischemic Stroke Investigators 2000).

The lack of effect of about 50 neuroprotectants that have been studied in clinical trials (Kidwell et al. 2001) has been explained by the multitude of pathways in the pathophysiology of stroke. In this view, each pathway contributes a little to the ischemic damage but not enough to see a clear effect when it is inhibited. The logical response to this problem would be to interfere with two or more pathogenic mechanisms at the same time. A combination of compounds might be effective although the individual compound has no effect when tested alone. Although this logic is intriguing, it might be difficult to test in the clinic. Pharmacodynamic, pharmacokinetic, and regulatory problems have to be solved before combination therapies could be tested. Moreover, pharmaceutical companies might not be interested in providing financial support if they do not hold the patent for all compounds to be tested.

The situation is different with rt-PA. After the FDA and other national regulatory agencies have approved rt-PA for routine use in acute stroke, the next step is to test rt-PA in combination with neuroprotective compounds (Grotta 2001; Lyden et al. 2001). Therefore, novel neuroprotectants have to be safe in combination with thrombolysis.

11.3 Patient Population

It is likely that the pathophysiology of lacunar, embolic, or hemorrhagic strokes differs. The success of experimental animal studies with a well-defined hypoperfusion in a single vascular territory has suggested that it might be favorable to limit the inclusion criteria in clinical studies to defined vascular territories. This notion was further supported by the post hoc analysis of the CLAS study that suggested that only patients with a large cortical infarct, a total anterior circulation stroke (TACS), would profit (Lyden et al. 2001). However, a follow-up investigation of these patients (CLASS-I) could not validate this hypothesis (Lyden et al. 2002). In CLASS and CLASS-I, selection of patients with TACS was based on clinical grounds and included patients with higher cortical dysfunction plus homonymous visual field defect plus limb weakness and an NIHSS of more than 3. A similar classification system known as Oxfordshire system to subgroup strokes on clinical grounds was shown to have some predictive value for the natural history of strokes (Bamford et al. 1991). So far, only a third of all controlled trials have specified a specific territory. Inclusion of strokes with a defined subset of stroke mechanisms has been even rarer (Kidwell et al. 2001). This is in part due to technical problems. Subgrouping using e.g., the TOAST criteria, often relies on additional investigations that are not readily available upon inclusion of patients (Adams et al. 1993). However, nowadays information on the presence of persisting vascular occlusion is becoming more and more available in the acute situation. Sonography and MR angiography allow the quick identification of occluded vessels. Although it seems logical to include this information into therapeutic considerations concerning thrombolysis (Schellinger et al. 2003), its value for therapeutic decisions has not been tested prospectively in controlled studies so far.

For neuroprotective and anti-inflammatory strategies there are even less pathophysiological approaches to identify the target stroke population that would benefit most. One obvious subgroup with a bad prognosis are those patients with elevated body temperature (Reith et al. 1996). However, it is unclear whether lowering body temperature to normothermia improves the prognosis. Nevertheless, due to the ease of this intervention most experts recommend antipyretic treatment in stroke patients with fever (Hacke et al. 2000). Beyond temperature there are several humoral markers of an acute inflammatory reaction in stroke patients. The acute phase proteins C-reactive protein (CRP) and fibrinogen are well-established markers of the inflammatory reaction that have a clear predictive value concerning the prognosis (Di Napoli et al. 2001 a, b). The acute phase reaction is directed by the cytokine interleukin-6 (IL-6). In acute stroke IL-6 serum concentrations rise rapidly. Indeed, experimental work shows that IL-6 is involved in stroke pathophysiology (Herrmann et al. 2003). While many other cytokines exert only paracrine effects in the direct vicinity of their production, IL-6 has also humoral properties. It stimulates the synthesis of acute phase proteins in the liver. Therefore, measurement of IL-6 in venous blood is dealing not with a spill-over but with an effective compartment. The IL-6 induction not only reflects the infarct size, but is also under genetic control (Acalovschi et al. 2003). Patients with a special haplotype of the IL-6 promoter mount a smaller increase of IL-6 serum concentrations in stroke. Thus, measurement of IL-6 in venous blood might lead to the early identification of stroke patients at risk of a severe inflammatory reaction. When the genetics of the inflammatory reaction in stroke will be better understood, it might be possible to define the patient population that will benefit most from anti-inflammatory therapies.

11.4 Time Window

In the last decades the time window in which patients were enrolled into clinical trials after onset of stroke has changed considerably (Kidwell et al. 2001). However, even in the last 5 years of the twentieth century the median time window for neuroprotective trials was 12 h. This is in clear contrast to experimental studies. In animals, the effect of neuroprotective agents and of thrombolytic agents on infarct size is time-dependent: early initiation of treatment works best; and benefit is progressively – and eventually totally – lost with increasing delay of time of first treatment (Jonas et al. 2001). In the lab, only very few compounds exert a protective effect beyond a time window of 6 h after onset of ischemia. This explains why clinical effects have above all been observed within a 3-h time window (Ninds Rt-Pa Stroke Study Group 1995). However, in clinical practice it is often not possible to start treatment within 3 h. This has motivated constant attempts to extend the time window. In April 2003, ECASS III will be launched; it will test the effect of thrombolysis in a dose of 0.9 mg/kg body weight between 3 and 4 h after onset of symptoms. Other trials that include patients beyond the 3-h time window are employing new MR technology (DIAS, Epiteth, Defuse). These studies rely on the hypothesis that patient subgroups who are likely to benefit from thrombolytic therapy can be identified based on a combination of blood flow parameters and an assessment of the degree of early ischemic brain injury – variables for which the MRI techniques of DWI and PWI are extremely sensitive.

11.5 Outcome Measures

Neurologic outcome can be scored by various scales. An overview is provided at the following website: http://www.strokecenter.org/trials/scales/scales-overview.htm. Most popular are scales of the neurologic deficit such as the NIH stroke scale (NIHSS), scales of global disability such as the modified Rankin scale (mRS), or scales of activities of daily living such as the Barthel score (BI; Rankin 1957; Bonita and Beaglehole 1988; Van Swieten et al. 1988; Brott et al.

Table 1. Time window of recent and future stroke trials

Trial name	Time window	Inclusion criteria
ECASS III	3–4 h	Clinical + CT
AbBEST	6 h	Clinical + CT
Repinotan	6 h (3 h cotreatment with rt-PA possible)	Clinical + CT
EPITETH, Defuse	3–6 h	Clinical + MRI
DIAS	3–9 h	Clinical + MRI
AbBEST II	3–5 h	Clinical + CT

1989). All three are quickly applied within a few minutes but lack sensitivity with strokes in several vascular territories such as the brain stem. Experience in ECASS I has suggested that it is better to dichotomize the modified Rankin scale and the Barthel index than to compare median levels (Hacke et al. 1998). Most recent studies define a favorable outcome as a score of 0 or 1 on mRS, a score of 95 or 100 on BI, and a score of 0 or 1 on NIHSS.

The interindividual variation of stroke scores at the time of inclusion into clinical trials is tremendous. Moreover, it is obvious that the early deficit predicts the outcome even if an effective therapy is installed. A patient with an NIHSS of 15 at inclusion into the study is less likely to have a favorable outcome as defined by a mRS of 0 than a patient with an NIHSS of 6. To adjust for this point the definition of a favorable outcome in AbBEST I was dependent on the initial deficit. The frequency of responders to therapy may have a lower variation than the traditional uniform definition of a favorable outcome. In AbBEST I this analysis proved to be very sensitive and yielded a significant result. However, it was only a prespecified secondary endpoint. In AbBEST II it will be the primary endpoint.

Another way to evaluate the individual improvement or deterioration is MRI. Diffusion weighted imaging (DWI) can be a surrogate marker of clinically meaningful lesion progression in stroke trials (Warach et al. 2000). The lesion can be detected very early after onset of symptoms. The combination of DWI and perfusion weighted imaging (PWI) allows an early evaluation of tissue that is hypoperfused but not yet irreversibly damaged (Schellinger et al. 2001).

This part of the lesion can be potentially saved. The DIAS trial uses this approach. Based on a percentage change in the PWI volume at 4–8 h post-treatment, a 30.7% median reduction in the PWI volume could be shown for desmoteplase compared to 7.2% for placebo.

Humoral surrogate parameters for cerebral ischemia are neuron-specific enolase (NSE) and S-100B. While NSE is a predominantly neuronal protein, S-100B is mainly released from astrocytes. Both proteins correlate with the infarct volume and the clinical outcome of stroke patients. However, the strength of these markers probably lies not in the evaluation of the infarct size, which is easily measured by radiologic means, but in the differential analysis of neuronal and astrocytic function. This approach has suggested that the AMPA antagonist ZK200775 worsens the neurologic deficit after acute stroke through glial toxicity (Elting et al. 2002).

In conclusion, there is no best endpoint. Therefore, most clinical trials use a combination of several endpoints. To improve the possibility of a positive trial result, a clinically relevant, easily performed score such as the mRS using a dichotomized statistical endpoint is preferred. Another question is the time point for the evaluation of the patient outcome. As a compromise 90 days are most widely used.

11.6 Number of Patients

Most neuroprotective trials to date have been powered to detect effects on the order of an absolute risk reduction of 10%. However, a 10% effect might be too optimistic. Such optimism is nourished by large effects in animal models and by the extrapolation from small phase II trials. For various reasons phase II trials may overestimate the efficacy of interventions (Samsa and Matchar 2001). A typical trial of an acute stroke tends to be on the "steep part of the power curve." An overestimation of the efficacy leads to a serious reduction in statistical power. Thrombolysis achieves 12% absolute improvement in independence (Lees 2002). Possibly neuroprotection is less effective. But due to the enormous costs of rehabilitation or lifetime care after stroke even a small reduction in the frequency of disability after stroke might be cost effective and of functional significance for the individual patient (Fagan et al. 1998; Caro and Huybrechts 1999; Samsa and Matchar 2001). If the actual improvement in good outcomes associated with neuroprotective treatment is 5%, a sample size of about 1,500 patients is needed for a power of 0.8. Usual patient numbers in former neuroprotective trials were, however, significantly smaller. In the clomethiazole trial 680 patients were included, in the tirilazad trial only 565 patients, and in the lubeluzole trial 368 patients. This reduced the power of these studies to a level of 0.5–0.3.

The number of patients needed for an informative trial is also influenced by the variation of the outcome parameter and the selection of patients. Population heterogeneity not only increases the variation of the outcome parameter, but is also afflicted with the possibility that the tested compound does not target all relevant mechanisms. It has been estimated that in two large neuroprotective trials, CLASS and GAIN-I, only between 20% to 50% of patients had a form of stroke that was a target of neuroprotective treatment (Muir 2002). However, this estimation is questionable as the pathophysiology of lacunar strokes is not clear enough to allow definite conclusions whether neuroprotective strategies would work.

11.7 Conclusion

Flaws in the design of early clinical trials in acute stroke contributed to their failure. Improvement of study design and the advent of new technology (e.g., MRI) hold the promise to establish neuroprotection in the clinic.

References

The Abciximab in Ischemic Stroke Investigators (2000) Abciximab in acute ischemic stroke: a randomized, double-blind, placebo-controlled, dose-escalation study. Stroke 31:601–609

Acalovschi D, Wiest T, Hartmann M, Farahmi M, Mansmann U, Auffarth GU, Grau AJ, Green F, Grond-Ginsbach C Schwaninger M (2003) Multiple levels of regulation of the interleukin-6 system in stroke. Stroke 34:1864–1870

Adams HP Jr, Bendixen BH, Kappelle LJ, Biller J, Love BB, Gordon DL Marsh EE 3rd (1993) Classification of subtype of acute ischemic stroke. Definitions for use in a multicenter clinical trial. TOAST. Trial of Org 10172 in Acute Stroke Treatment. Stroke 24:35–41

Bamford J, Sandercock P, Dennis M, Burn J, Warlow C (1991) Classification and natural history of clinically identifiable subtypes of cerebral infarction. Lancet 337:1521–1526

Bonita R, Beaglehole R (1988) Recovery of motor function after stroke. Stroke 19:1497–1500

Brott T, Adams HP Jr, Olinger CP, Marler JR, Barsan WG, Biller J, Spilker J, Holleran R, Eberle R, Hertzberg V, et al (1989) Measurements of acute cerebral infarction: a clinical examination scale. Stroke 20:864–870

Caro JJ, Huybrechts KF (1999) Stroke treatment economic model (STEM): predicting long-term costs from functional status. Stroke 30:2574–2579

Dawson DA, Wadsworth G, Palmer AM (2001) A comparative assessment of the efficacy and side-effect liability of neuroprotective compounds in experimental stroke. Brain Res 892:344–350

Di Napoli M, Papa F, Bocola V (2001a) C-reactive protein in ischemic stroke: an independent prognostic factor. Stroke 32:917–924

Di Napoli M, Papa F, Bocola V (2001b) Prognostic influence of increased C-reactive protein and fibrinogen levels in ischemic stroke. Stroke 32:133–138

Elting JW, Sulter GA, Kaste M, Lees KR, Diener HC, Hommel M, Versavel M, Teelken AW, De Keyser J (2002) AMPA antagonist ZK200775 in patients with acute ischemic stroke: possible glial cell toxicity detected by monitoring of S-100B serum levels. Stroke 33:2813–2818

Fagan SC, Morgenstern LB, Petitta A, Ward RE, Tilley BC, Marler JR, Levine SR, Broderick JP, Kwiatkowski TG, Frankel M, Brott TG, Walker MD (1998) Cost-effectiveness of tissue plasminogen activator for acute ischemic stroke. NINDS rt-PA Stroke Study Group. Neurology 50:883–890

Furlan A, Higashida R, Wechsler L, Gent M, Rowley H, Kase C, Pessin M, Ahuja A, Callahan F, Clark WM, Silver F, Rivera F (1999) Intra-arterial prourokinase for acute ischemic stroke. The PROACT II study: a randomized controlled trial. Prolyse in acute cerebral thromboembolism. JAMA 282:2003–2011

Grotta J (2001) Combination therapy stroke trial: recombinant tissue-type plasminogen activator with/without lubeluzole. Cerebrovasc Dis 12:258–263

Hacke W, Bluhmki E, Steiner T, Tatlisumak T, Mahagne MH, Sacchetti ML, Meier D (1998) Dichotomized efficacy end points and global end-point analysis applied to the ECASS intention-to-treat data set: post hoc analysis of ECASS I. Stroke 29:2073–2075

Hacke W, Kaste M, Olsen TS, Bogousslavsky J, Orgogozo JM, Committee ftEE (2000) Acute treatment of ischemic stroke. Cerebrovasc Dis 10 [Suppl 3]:22–33

Herrmann O, Tarabin V, Suzuki S, Attigah N, Prinz S, Schneider A, Coserea I, Monyer H, Brombacher F, Schwaninger M (2003) Regulation of body temperature and neuroprotection by endogenous interleukin-6 in focal cerebral ischemia. J Cereb Blood Flow Metab 23:406–415

Jonas S, Aiyagari V, Vieira D, Figueroa M (2001) The failure of neuronal protective agents versus the success of thrombolysis in the treatment of ischemic stroke. The predictive value of animal models. Ann N Y Acad Sci 939:257–267

Kay R, Wong KS, Yu YL, Chan YW, Tsoi TH, Ahuja AT, Chan FL, Fong KY, Law CB, Wong A (1995) Low-molecular-weight heparin for the treatment of acute ischemic stroke. N Engl J Med 333:1588–1593

Kidwell CS, Liebeskind DS, Starkman S, Saver JL (2001) Trends in acute ischemic stroke trials through the 20th century. Stroke 32:1349–1359

Lees KR (2002) Neuroprotection is unlikely to be effective in humans using current trial design: an opposing view. Stroke 33:308–309

Lyden P, Jacoby M, Schim J, Albers G, Mazzeo P, Ashwood T, Nordlund A, Odergren T (2001) The Clomethiazole Acute Stroke Study in tissue-type plasminogen activator-treated stroke (CLASS-T): final results. Neurology 57:1199–1205

Lyden P, Shuaib A, Ng K, Levin K, Atkinson RP, Rajput A, Wechsler L, Ashwood T, Claesson L, Odergren T, Salazar-Grueso E (2002) Clomethiazole Acute Stroke Study in ischemic stroke (CLASS-I): final results. Stroke 33:122–128

Muir KW (2002) Heterogeneity of stroke pathophysiology and neuroprotective clinical trial design. Stroke 33:1545–1550

NINDS rt-PA Stroke Study Group (1995) Tissue plasminogen activator for acute ischemic stroke. N Engl J Med 333:1581–1587

Rankin J (1957) Cerebral vascular accidents in patients over the age of 60. Scott Med J 2:200–215

Reith J, Jorgensen H, Pedersen P, Nakayama H, Raaschou H, Jeppesen L, Olsen T (1996) Body temperature in acute stroke: relation to stroke severity, infarct size, mortality, and outcome. Lancet 347:422–425

Samsa GP, Matchar DB (2001) Have randomized controlled trials of neuroprotective drugs been underpowered? An illustration of three statistical principles. Stroke 32:669–674

Schellinger PD, Fiebach JB, Jansen O, Ringleb PA, Mohr A, Steiner T, Heiland S, Schwab S, Pohlers O, Ryssel H, Orakcioglu B, Sartor K, Hacke W (2001) Stroke magnetic resonance imaging within 6 h after onset of hyperacute cerebral ischemia. Ann Neurol 49:460–469

Schellinger PD, Fiebach JB, Hacke W (2003) Imaging-based decision making in thrombolytic therapy for ischemic stroke: present status. Stroke 34:575–583

Sherman DG, Atkinson RP, Chippendale T, Levin KA, Ng K, Futrell N, Hsu CY, Levy DE (2000) Intravenous ancrod for treatment of acute ischemic stroke. The STAT study: a randomized controlled trial. Stroke Treatment with Ancrod Trial. JAMA 283:2395–2403

van Swieten JC, Koudstaal PJ, Visser MC, Schouten HJ, van Gijn J (1988) Interobserver agreement for the assessment of handicap in stroke patients. Stroke 19:604–607

Warach S, Pettigrew LC, Dashe JF, Pullicino P, Lefkowitz DM, Sabounjian L, Harnett K, Schwiderski U, Gammans R (2000) Effect of citicoline on ischemic lesions as measured by diffusion-weighted magnetic resonance imaging. Citicoline 010 Investigators. Ann Neurol 48:713–722

Subject Index

Ernst Schering Research Foundation Workshop

Editors: Günter Stock
Monika Lessl

Vol. 1 (1991): Bioscience ⇋ Societly Workshop Report
Editors: D.J. Roy, B.E. Wynne, R.W. Old

Vol. 2 (1991): Round Table Discussion on Bioscience ⇋ Society
Editor: J.J. Cherfas

Vol. 3 (1991): Excitatory Amino Acids and Second Messenger Systems
Editors: V.I. Teichberg, L. Turski

Vol. 4 (1992): Spermatogenesis – Fertilization – Contraception
Editors: E. Nieschlag, U.-F. Habenicht

Vol. 5 (1992): Sex Steroids and the Cardiovascular System
Editors: P. Ramwell, G. Rubanyi, E. Schillinger

Vol. 6 (1993): Transgenic Animals as Model Systems for Human Diseases
Editors: E.F. Wagner, F. Theuring

Vol. 7 (1993): Basic Mechanisms Controlling Term and Preterm Birth
Editors: K. Chwalisz, R.E. Garfield

Vol. 8 (1994): Health Care 2010
Editors: C. Bezold, K. Knabner

Vol. 9 (1994): Sex Steroids and Bone
Editors: R. Ziegler, J. Pfeilschifter, M. Bräutigam

Vol. 10 (1994): Nongenotoxic Carcinogenesis
Editors: A. Cockburn, L. Smith

Vol. 11 (1994): Cell Culture in Pharmaceutical Research
Editors: N.E. Fusenig, H. Graf

Vol. 12 (1994): Interactions Between Adjuvants, Agrochemical
and Target Organisms
Editors: P.J. Holloway, R.T. Rees, D. Stock

Vol. 13 (1994): Assessment of the Use of Single Cytochrome
P450 Enzymes in Drug Research
Editors: M.R. Waterman, M. Hildebrand

Vol. 14 (1995): Apoptosis in Hormone-Dependent Cancers
Editors: M. Tenniswood, H. Michna

Vol. 15 (1995): Computer Aided Drug Design in Industrial Research
Editors: E.C. Herrmann, R. Franke

Vol. 16 (1995): Organ-Selective Actions of Steroid Hormones
Editors: D.T. Baird, G. Schütz, R. Krattenmacher

Vol. 17 (1996): Alzheimer's Disease
Editors: J.D. Turner, K. Beyreuther, F. Theuring

Vol. 18 (1997): The Endometrium as a Target for Contraception
Editors: H.M. Beier, M.J.K. Harper, K. Chwalisz

Vol. 19 (1997): EGF Receptor in Tumor Growth and Progression
Editors: R.B. Lichtner, R.N. Harkins

Vol. 20 (1997): Cellular Therapy
Editors: H. Wekerle, H. Graf, J.D. Turner

Vol. 21 (1997): Nitric Oxide, Cytochromes P 450,
and Sexual Steroid Hormones
Editors: J.R. Lancaster, J.F. Parkinson

Vol. 22 (1997): Impact of Molecular Biology
and New Technical Developments in Diagnostic Imaging
Editors: W. Semmler, M. Schwaiger

Vol. 23 (1998): Excitatory Amino Acids
Editors: P.H. Seeburg, I. Bresink, L. Turski

Vol. 24 (1998): Molecular Basis of Sex Hormone Receptor Function
Editors: H. Gronemeyer, U. Fuhrmann, K. Parczyk

Vol. 25 (1998): Novel Approaches to Treatment of Osteoporosis
Editors: R.G.G. Russell, T.M. Skerry, U. Kollenkirchen

Vol. 26 (1998): Recent Trends in Molecular Recognition
Editors: F. Diederich, H. Künzer

Vol. 27 (1998): Gene Therapy
Editors: R.E. Sobol, K.J. Scanlon, E. Nestaas, T. Strohmeyer

Vol. 28 (1999): Therapeutic Angiogenesis
Editors: J.A. Dormandy, W.P. Dole, G.M. Rubanyi

Vol. 29 (2000): Of Fish, Fly, Worm and Man
Editors: C. Nüsslein-Volhard, J. Krätzschmar

Vol. 30 (2000): Therapeutic Vaccination Therapy
Editors: P. Walden, W. Sterry, H. Hennekes

Vol. 31 (2000): Advances in Eicosanoid Research
Editors: C.N. Serhan, H.D. Perez

Vol. 32 (2000): The Role of Natural Products in Drug Discovery
Editors: J. Mulzer, R. Bohlmann

Supplement 1 (1994): Molecular and Cellular Endocrinology of the Testis
Editors: G. Verhoeven, U.-F. Habenicht

Supplement 2 (1997): Signal Transduction in Testicular Cells
Editors: V. Hansson, F.O. Levy, K. Taskén

Supplement 3 (1998): Testicular Function:
From Gene Expression to Genetic Manipulation
Editors: M. Stefanini, C. Boitani, M. Galdieri, R. Geremia,
F. Palombi

Supplement 4 (2000): Hormone Replacement Therapy
and Osteoporosis
Editors: J. Kato, H. Minaguchi, Y. Nishino

Supplement 5 (1999): Interferon: The Dawn of Recombinant
Protein Drugs
Editors: J. Lindenmann, W.D. Schleuning

Supplement 6 (2000): Testis, Epididymis and Technologies
in the Year 2000
Editors: B. Jégou, C. Pineau, J. Saez

Supplement 7 (2001): New Concepts in Pathology and
Treatment of Autoimmune Disorders
Editors: P. Pozzilli, C. Pozzilli, J.-F. Kapp

Supplement 8 (2001): New Pharmacological Approaches
to Reproductive Health and Healthy Ageing
Editors: W.-K. Raff, M.F. Fathalla, F. Saad

Supplement 9 (2002): Testicular Tangrams
Editors: F.F.G. Rommerts, K.J. Teerds

Supplement 10 (2002): Die Architektur des Lebens
Editors: G. Stock, M. Lessl

This series will be available on request from
Ernst Schering Research Foundation, 13342 Berlin, Germany